I0481362

CHOLESTEROL CONSPIRACY and SCANDALOUS LIES

Cholesterol Is The Mother Of all nutrients and We Will Die without It

Cholesterol Is Not Your Enemy your Brain and Cells need it

Why Then So Many Scandalous Lies about Cholesterol

Lower Your Cholesterol Naturally without Serious Side effects

Serious Health Hazards of cholesterol Lowering Statin Drugs

Cholesterol is Not The Villain It is The Oxidation of Cholesterol

Dr. Arta Tran Dash, M.Sc., M. S., Ph. D.

Retired Professor

INTRODUCTION

CHOLESTEROL

What is Cholesterol?

Cholesterol is a white soft, fat-like, waxy substance found in the bloodstream and in all cells of our body. It occurs naturally in every cell or membrane everywhere in the body, including the brain, nerves, muscles, skin, liver, intestines, and heart. Cholesterol is an essential part of a healthy body and the body uses it to produce cell membranes, several important hormones (e.g. testosterone, progesterone, estrogen, DHEA, etc.), vitamin D, and bile acids that help digest fats

Your Brain Needs Cholesterol

Cholesterol is vitally important for brain function. While your brain represents about 2-3% of your total body weight, 25% of the cholesterol in your body is found in your brain, where it plays important roles in such things as membrane function, acts as powerful brain antioxidant, and serves as the raw material from which we are able to make things like progesterone, estrogen, cortisol, testosterone and vitamin D3.

25% Of The Body's Cholesterol Is In The Brain, Keeping You Alzheimer's-Free

Furthermore, we summarize below why Cholesterol is part of your body...

- Your cells' walls are made of it.
- Cholesterol is a building block of cell membranes
- Your brain is made of it
- Vital hormones, like testosterone, progesterone, estrogen,
- cortisol are made from it as mentioned above.
- Your body can't digest fat without it.
- Your body can't produce vitamin D without it.

Cholesterol Is Not Your Enmey

Most people are told cardiovascular diseases are due to cholesterol clumping together to form build ups that block the flow of blood.

Cholesterol is a **vital nutrient** your body uses to repair rips, tears, or growths in the walls of your blood vessels. When damage occurs, cholesterol flowing in the blood stops to coat and repair the damaged area. As more layers of cholesterol are added for healing, a bulge of cholesterol is formed. Imagine what will happen to your blood vessels if cholesterol does not repair the rips, tears and growths in the walls of your blood vessels.

*Unfortunately, these **bulges** are what have given cholesterol its bad reputation*

Cholesterol Lowering Drugs (Statin drugs)

The following is a list of cholesterol lowering drugs.

- Statins: alorvastatin (Lipitor), Simvastatin (Zocor), Lovastatin (Mevacor), Pravastatin (Pravachol), Rosuvastatin (Crestor), and others

- Bile acid Sequestrants
- Nicotinic Acid
- Fibrates
- Hormone Replacement Therapy

Serious Side Effects of Statin Drugs

Any patient taking these drugs should be regularly monitored by his physician for any serious side effects. These drugs have potentially harmful side effects, such as upset stomach, gas, constipation, abdominal pain or cramps, nausea, diarrhea. Other symptoms are: abnormalities in blood tests of the liver. You may also experience symptoms, such as muscle soreness, joint pain and weakness or brown urine, contact your doctor right away. These drugs eventually may lead to liver damage

Increased blood sugar or risk of type 2 diabetes

Neurological side effects: memory loss or confusion, dementia, cognitive damage

Copyrights@2017 by Arta Tran Dash, M.Sc., M.S., Ph. D.,

 All rights reserved. Reproduction or storage in a retrieval system or data base or transmission in any form or by any means, electrical, mechanical, photocopying or otherwise are forbidden, without the permission of the author.

LOKA SAMASTA SUKHINO BHABANTU

(Let Each And Every Person In The Universe Be Hale and Hearty)

VEDAS

DISCLAIMER

This book is not intended to diagnose, treat or replace the service of a doctor. If you have any health conditions or are under a doctor's care, you must consult your physician or a healthcare professional before you apply any of the recommendations set forth in the pages of this book.

All information available in this book is for educational purposes only, and none of the stated products have been FDA approved. Any application of the recommendations mentioned in this book is at the readers' discretion and sole risk.

The publication is offered "as is" without warranty of any kind either expressed or implied, including but not limited to, the implied warranties of merchantability, suitability for a particular purpose or non-infringement. Descriptions of or reference to products or publications does not imply endorsement of that product or publication.

Here is how you can use the information in this book to improve your health and wellness. Being Empowered with these powerful armies of information, and the knowledge gathered from it, you would be able to discuss your health problems with a healthcare professional and design a regimen that is conducive to your health and well being, instead of just being drugged to death and suffer from lethal side effects of these drugs, causing serious debilitating, chronic diseases, even death.

If you find your physician is unwilling to discuss the issue, find another physician or a healthcare professional who is more sensitive to your wish and willing to take the time to listen to you for your well being. You need to know all your options before embarking on a particular regimen or a procedure.

TABLE OF CONTENTS

CHAPTER ONE

- what is cholesterol?
- Cholesterol is vital for functioning of the cells
- your brain needs cholesterol
- testosterone, progesterone, estrogen
- coronary heart disease
- Cholesterol is building block of your cells

CHAPTER TWO

- Where do we get our cholesterol?
- Low density lipoprotein (LDL), bad cholesterol
- High density lipoprotein (HDL), good cholesterol
- Lp(a) cholesterol

CHAPTER THREE

- Triglycerides
- Triglyceridenia
- Cirrhosis (liver disease
- Classification of triglyceride levels
- How to lower triglyceride levels
- apoB and apoA cholesterol particles
- reference ranges for apoB and apoA
- the ratio apoB/apoA

CHAPTER FOUR

- where the body gets cholesterol?
- what your cholesterol levels mean?
- desirable cholesterol levels
- LDL cholesterol level at which one should consider drug therapy
- cholesterol ratio
- cholesterol in women and children
- lipid peroxidation

CHAPTER FIVE

- cholesterol conspiracy and scandalous lies
- free radicals and oxidation of cholesterol
- cholesterol is not the villain, it is oxidation of cholesterol
- cholesterol oxidation: health hazards and antioxidants to rescue
- antioxidants: vitaminsA, B's, C, E, D3, CoQ10 and PQQ, alpha lipoic acid, glutathione, resveratrol
- omega - 3 fatty acids

CHAPTER SIX

- cholesterol is not your enemy
- real cause of circulation problem is calcium
- scandalous lies about cholesterol
- fast and fried foods
- saturated fats, trans fats
- overweight and sedentary life style
- testing procedures

CHAPTER SEVEN

- fiber and foods can help lower cholesterol
- health benefits of fiber
- soluble and insoluble fiber
- short chain fatty acids
- tips for adding more fiber to your diet
- fiber inulin
- health benefits of fiber inulin
- oats vs oat bran, and heart disease
- diabetes

CHAPTER EIGHT

- treatments to lower cholesterol levels
- foods recommended
- avocado
- apple
- cholesterol and fats
- foods to avoid
- butter vs margarine

CPAPTER NINE

- cholesterol beyond hype
- cholesterol is the mother of all nutrients
- triglyceride
- homocysteine
- C-reactive Protein (CRP)

CHAPTER TEN

- Cholesterol lowering Statin drugs and Side effects
- serious side effects of statin drugs
- increased blood sugar or risk of Type 2 diabetes
- memory loss, confusion
- dementia and cognitive damage
- risk of peripheral Neuropathy
- muscle cramps
- depletion of CoQ10, the heart tonic

CHAPTER ELEVEN

- lower cholesterol levels naturally without side effects
- vitamins C, E, D3, EPA & DHA, CoQ10 & PQQ, lipoic acid
- omega – 3 fatty acids
- glucamannana
- aged garlic extract
- policosanol
- guggul
- niacin
- Arjuna
- Beta sitosterol

CHAPTER TWELEVE

- Therapeutic and anti-aging nutrients
- unpasteurized raw honey
- apple cider vinegar
- hair care
- rooibos tea health benefits

- rooinos tea ease inflammation
- health benefits of ginger
- ginger increases heart's strength, and
  helps produce significant reduction in blood platelets clumping
- beta sitosterol

CHAPTER THIRTEEN

- practice meditations, living in present, and selfawareness
- practice Kriya yoga
- listen to the voice in your head
- self realization
- aromatherapy
- air freshener
- ingredients in air refreshener

CHAPTER ONE

CHOLESTEROL

What is Cholesterol?

Cholesterol is a white soft, fat-like, waxy substance found in the bloodstream and in all cells of our body. It occurs naturally in every cell or membrane everywhere in the body, including the brain, nerves, muscles, skin, liver, intestines, and heart. Cholesterol is an essential part of a healthy body and the body uses it to produce cell membranes, several important hormones (e.g. testosterone, progesterone, estrogen, DHEA, etc.), vitamin D, and bile acids that help digest fats. It takes only a small amount of cholesterol to meet these needs. Thus, cholesterol is not all that bad, since it is vital for proper functioning of the cells, making hormones, used in myelin sheath formation (the membrane covering around nerves.)

Your Brain Needs Cholesterol

Cholesterol is vitally important for brain function. While your brain represents about 2-3% of your total body weight, 25% of the cholesterol in your body is found in your brain, where it plays important roles in such things as membrane function, acts as powerful brain antioxidant, and serves as the raw material from which we are able to make things like progesterone, estrogen, cortisol, testosterone and vitamin D3.

25% Of The Body's Cholesterol Is In The Brain, Keeping You Alzheimer's-Free

Our brain is 60 percent fat, with over 25 percent of that being cholesterol. Most of the cholesterol in the brain is produced in the hypothalamus itself, establishing cholesterol as an integral part of our brain. It is also needed for proper functioning of the brain. Thus, without cholesterol you will die.

Furthermore, we summarize below why Cholesterol is part of your body...

- Your cells' walls are made of it.
- Cholesterol is a building block of cell membranes
- Your brain is made of it.
- Vital hormones, like testosterone, progesterone, estrogen,
- cortisol are made from it as mentioned above.

- Your body can't digest fat without it.
- Your body can't produce vitamin D without it.
-

It's very foolish to declare war on a part of your body. You can't win.

However, problems arise when we have too much cholesterol in the bloodstream—hypercholesterolemia—circulating through our veins and arteries. This excess cholesterol deposited in the arteries, including the coronary arteries—a primary factor for coronary heart disease leading to heart attack and stroke. Too much of these deposits in the arteries inhibit the circulation and may also cause gallstones, impotence, high blood pressure, and loss of mental acuity.

CHAPTER TWO

WHERE DO WE GET OUR CHOLESTEROL?

We get cholesterol from two sources: our body produces most of it and the rest we get from cholesterol in animal products that we consume, such as meats, eggs, fish, butter, cheese and whole milk. Foods from plants: Fruits and vegetables do not contain cholesterol. Foods from other sources that may not contain animal products may consist of saturated fats, trans-fats, and hydrogenated fats and oils that make the body produce excess cholesterol. Processed foods, including deli, not only contain bad fats, but also contain chemicals (e.g., nitrates, aspartame) that may make the body produce excess cholesterol and possibly cause cancer. See more detailed discussion in a later section.

As we know, oil and water don't mix. This implies that cholesterol and other fats cannot dissolve in blood. Thus, they have to be carried to and from the cells through a special medium called lipoproteins. Differently expressed, cholesterol must be attached to transport molecules lipoproteins to remain in circulation. Although, there are many different kinds of lipoproteins, we only need to know two kinds: **low-density lipoprotein or (LDL),** known as **bad** cholesterol, and **high-density lipoprotein or HDL** known as **good** cholesterol. We shall discuss them in detail below.

About LDL, HDL, and the Difference between them

LDL Cholesterol (Bad Cholesterol)

Low-density-lipoprotein (LDL) is the main carrier of cholesterol in the blood. It carries cholesterol from the liver, where it is produced, to the cells and tissues in the body that need it. On the other hand, high-density-lipoprotein (HDL) carries cholesterol from the arteries to the liver for metabolism and excretion or to be reprocessed. Under ideal conditions lipoproteins keep cholesterol levels under control. However, this amazingly orchestrated system can be overwhelmed when the body produces too much cholesterol which HDL is unable to sweep away. After the cells use whatever they need, HDLs remove some of it, the remaining cholesterol simply stays in the blood. This creates serious health problems.

 If excessive LDL cholesterol circulates in the blood, it can slowly build up deposits in the arteries feeding the heart and brain. Furthermore, if cholesterol (especially LDL) gets oxidized by highly reactive oxygen species (called free radicals, see later) and attaches to the arterial walls itself, setting the stage for the onslaught of inflamed arteries.

This chronic inflammation leads to a further buildup of cholesterol deposits that combined with other substances forms plaque (a thick hard deposits) on the interior walls of the arteries. This clogs the arteries leading to atherosclerosis (hardening of the arteries.) A clot (thrombus) that develops near plaque and blocks the narrowed artery can stop the blood flow to the heart muscle and produce a heart attack. A clot that stops blood flow to part of the brain can cause a stroke.

The condition that develops cholesterol buildup and deposits, which narrow the arteries and blocks the blood flow through them, is known as atherosclerosis or hardening of the arteries. It signals the onset of heart disease and left untreated may result in heart attack and stroke. This is why LDL is called **bad** cholesterol. A high level of LDL cholesterol (160 mg/dl and above) leads to an increased risk of heart attack and strokes. If you have problems, your total cholesterol levels should be less than 100 mg/dl. Here dl = deciliter.

HDL Cholesterol

HDL cholesterol is known as **good** cholesterol because of the following reasons. Roughly one-third to one forth of blood cholesterol is carried by HDL. As mentioned earlier, LDL transports cholesterol to the cells and tissues, whereas HDL carries cholesterol from the arterial walls and tissues back to the liver where it is metabolized and excreted through the bile. HDL also removes excess cholesterol from plaque and hence slows down its growth. Thus, one needs to maintain a high HDL cholesterol level and a low LDL cholesterol level to reduce the risk of heart disease and stroke. On the other hand a low HDL cholesterol level (less than 40 mg/dl in men, less than 50 mg/dl in women) signals a greater risk of heart disease and stroke. Here dl= deciliter.

These discussions lead to a new indicator that can predict the risk of heart disease with greater accuracy. This indicator is the important HDL-to-LDL (HDL/LDL) ratio that indicates whether cholesterol is being deposited into arteries and tissues or being broken down and excreted. The higher is this ratio (this means HDL cholesterol level is higher than the LDL cholesterol level), the lower is the risk of getting heart disease and stroke.

Indeed, research studies have shown that a I percent drop in the LDL (the ratio HDL/LDL becomes higher) cholesterol level, the risk for heart attack drops by two percent. On the other hand, a one percent increase in HDL (i.e, the ratio HDL/LDL gets higher) cholesterol levels reduces the risk for heart attack by 3 to 4 percent. This means, your HDL levels are more important than your total cholesterol levels. Thus, raising HDL cholesterol levels and simultaneously lowering LDL cholesterol levels make the ratio HDL/LDL higher and hence a greater protection against heart disease and stroke.

About Lp(a) Cholesterol

Lp(a) cholesterol is considered to be a genetic variation of LDL blood cholesterol. A high level of Lp(a) encourages fatty deposit buildups prematurely. The lesions in artery walls contain substances that may combine with Lp(a) contributing to fatty deposit buildups.

CHAPTER THREE

Triglycerides

Like cholesterol triglycerides are types of fats (lipids) present in blood plasma. They are essential for good health when present in ideal amounts. Triglycerides are responsible for 95 % of the body's fat tissues. People with high triglycerides generally have high LDL (bad) cholesterol and low HDL (good) cholesterol, and hence are in danger of getting heart attack or stroke.

Triglycerides in blood plasma are obtained from fats ingested from foods and the body manufactures it from other sources like carbohydrates. Calories taken from foods and not used immediately by tissues are converted to fat cells and stored. Hormones regulate the release of triglycerides from fat tissues to meet the body's requirements for energy between meals.

Excess triglyceride in the bloodstream is known as triglyceridemia. It is attributed to the onset of coronary artery diseases, such as hardening of arteries (atherosclerosis) and stroke. Abnormally, high triglyceride levels are normally consequences of a host of diseases and untreated conditions, such as cirrhosis (a liver disease), hypothyroidism (underactive thyroid), diabetes mellitus, pancreatitis ((inflammation of pancreas), and atherosclerosis. Studies have shown that high triglycerides levels are linked to an increased risk of strokes.

Studies also accounted for the fact that people with more than 200 mg of triglycerides per dl (deciliter) of blood were about 30 % more likely to have an ischemic stroke (mini stroke) or TIA (transitory ischemic attack, i.e., a brief interruption of blood flow to the brain) than people with lower levels of triglycerides.

At the very least, high triglyceride levels are a warning signal that a patient's cardiovascular health is at risk. People with this condition are usually advised (by their physicians) to take precaution in maintaining an ideal weight, getting adequate exercise, quitting smoking, regulating diabetes, insulin resistance and hypothyroidism, and consuming proper diet to protect their coronary health.

Classification of Triglyceride Levels

According to the US National Heart, Lung, and Blood Institute, the most current guide-line levels for triglycerides in milligrams per deciliter (mg/dl) are as follows.

- less than 150 mg/dl represents normal
- 150 to 199 mg/dl is considered border line
- 200 to 499 mg/dl is high, may require treatment in some people.
- 500 mg/dl or higher is considered very high. Persons with very high cholesterol need immediate treatment

Numerous studies, such as *Circulation*, 1997; 96:2520-2525; and *Circulation* 1998;17(11):1027-8. have shown that triglyceride levels in the blood may help predict the risk of heart attack as accurately as others, like blood fats LDL and HDL cholesterol levels. According to a report in a 1997 issue of *Circulation* mentioned above, high triglyceride level alone increased the risk of heart attack by 3-fold; and also people with the highest ratio of triglyceride to HDL cholesterol had a 16 times greater risk of heart attack than those with the lowest ratio of triglycerides to HDL. A Harvard study chronicled that the ratio of triglyceride to HDL was the strongest predictor of a heart attack, even more accurate than the LDL to HDL ratio.

How To Lower Triglyceride Lvels

High triglyceride levels are one of the easiest conditions that can be tackled with proper diet and exercise. Some of the culprits in elevating triglyceride levels are carbohydrates, simple sugars, sugars, grains, and lack of exercise.

The grains are rapidly metabolized to simple sugars. As studies suggest, this elevates the triglyceride levels in the blood. Sugars and grains require extra insulin secretion for metabolism, which stimulates the liver to produce more triglycerides. Instead of using drugs to lower triglyceride levels, it is safer just to markedly reduce altogether, if you have the condition, the intake of sugars and grains.

Elevated triglyceride levels in the blood are often found in overweight people. Even people who are not overweight may have fat deposits in the arteries as a result of insulin resistance. These triglyceride levels in the bloodstream do not directly come from dietary fats, instead they are produced in the liver from any excess sugar which has not been used for energy. See below for further recommendations.

- reduce or eliminate consumption of sugars, refined carbohydrates, pops, sweetened yogurt, cookies, desserts, candy, white bread, processed foods, fried foods, fast foods. Have whole fruit rather than juice Try brown rice, parboiled rice, quinoa, oat meal, barley.

- make every effort to maintain an ideal body weight. Even a modest weight loss of 5 to 10 pounds can be very beneficial.

- consume foods rich in beneficial fats. For instance, olive oil, coconut oil, avocado oil, avocado, peanuts, almonds, Brazil nuts, almonds, walnuts, sunflower seeds, and fatty fish like salmon, white fish, mackerel, sardines, and deep water fish. Note: oils, avocado, nuts are high in calories. If you have a weight problem, keep your potion sizes small.

- Study shows that coconut oil and avocado help reduce weight

- reduce or avoid saturated fats, hydrogenated fats, and trans-fats. Limit consumption of high fat diary product (i.e., cheese, ice cream,), high fat meats, most baked foods and pastries, French fries, doughnuts, muffins, bagels, and margarine.

- consume omega 3-fatty acids, monounsaturated and polyunsaturated fats.

- have a regular exercise regimen, and stop smoking.

About apoB and apoA-1 Cholesterol Particles

Apolipoprotein B (apoB) is a protein which is the primary component of low-density-cholesterol, LDL. Over 90 % of LDL cholesterol is composed of apoB. Furthermore, ApoB is responsible in transporting cholesterol to arteries and tissues. Although, it is unclear exactly what functional role it plays in LDL, it is the primary component and absolutely required for its formation. High apoB levels can lead to plaque formation, thereby increasing the risk of heart disease and stroke.

On other hand, apolipoprotein A1 (apoA1) is primarily found in HDL cholesterol and offers a protective shield against heart disease and stroke. Studies have shown that apoB level is a better marker than the total LDL cholesterol level. Besides LDL, apoB is also found in several other harmful cholesterols, such as very-low-density-lipoprotein (VLDL).

About APOA-1

The **APOA-1** gene provides instructions for making a protein called apolipoprotein A-I (apoA-I). ApoA-I is a component of high-density lipoprotein (HDL). HDL is a molecule that transports cholesterol and certain fats called phospholipids through the bloodstream from the body's tissues to the liver, where cholesterol and phospholipids are redistributed to other tissues or removed from the body.

ApoA-I attaches to cell membranes and promotes the movement of cholesterol and phospholipids from inside the cell to the outer surface, where these substances combine with apoA-I to form HDL. ApoA-I also triggers a reaction called cholesterol etherification that converts cholesterol to a form that can be fully integrated into HDL and transported through the bloodstream

A large study called AMORIS (apolipoprotein—related Mortality Risk)was conducted in Sweden involving 175,000 men and women where researchers measured the levels of apoA1 and apoB and also other lipids as well. They found that people at greatest risk of dying from a heart attack seem to have the highest ratio of apoB to apoA1 (apoB/apoA1). In this study, these newer markers were proven to be a better predictor of a heart attack than were the usual total HDL, LDL cholesterol, and triglycerides levels. Moreover, it was shown that the people with the highest aopB/apoA1 ratio had nearly four times the risk of fatal heart attack than those with the lowest ratio; and in women the relative risk was three-fold.

Reference Ranges For apoB, apoA-1 and The Ratio apoB/apoA-1

apoB reference range: 55-125 mg/dl

apoA1 reference range: 125-215 mg/dl

aopB/aopA1 reference range: 0.256-1.0

CHAPTER FOUR

WHERE DOES THE BODY GET CHOLESTEROL ?

WHAT ARE HEALTHY AND RISKY LEVELS

OF CHOLESTEROL AND TRIGLYCERIDES?

Where Does The Body Get Cholesterol?

We get cholesterol from two sources. Our body—mostly the liver produces cholesterol in varying degrees, ranging upto1000 milligrams a day. Typically the body makes all the cholesterol it needs. It only requires 10 percent of its cholesterol needs from dietary sources. This means that the treatment regimen for high cholesterol should be to control the dietary intake of cholesterol.

This means the Body only needs 10 % of cholesterol from food sources. Thus, we have to be careful as to what we eat. Unfortunately, North American foods are loaded with animal products, saturated fats, hydrogenated fats, trans-fats, and refined carbohydrates, processed foods, preservative chemicals which cause elevated cholesterol levels. Elevated cholesterol levels may also be caused by hereditary conditions and/or preexisting diseases, such as diabetes, insulin resistance, and syndrome X. Moreover, body accumulates cholesterol from intake of animal foods, especially meat, poultry, fish, seafood, egg yokes, processed meats (i.e., Deli, sausage, bacon, hot dogs) and dairy products. On the other hand, foods from plant sources,, such as fruits, vegetables, grains, nuts and seeds do not contain cholesterol.

An average North American man ingests roughly 337 milligram cholesterol per day, a woman about 217 milligrams. Ideally, some of the excess dietary cholesterol is generally eliminated by the liver. Yet the American Heart Association recommends that you restrict your average daily cholesterol intake to less than 300 milligrams a day, and if you have heart problems, limit your daily intake of cholesterol to 200 milligrams. If your cholesterol levels are high, just by reducing the consumption of dietary saturated fats, and trans fats, meats, egg yolk, carbohydrates, processed foods, you can significantly reduce your dietary cholesterol intake, and thus, this will enable you to significantly reduce your blood cholesterol levels.

Foods high in saturated fats and trans fats contain significant amounts of dietary cholesterol. In case you want further reduction of cholesterol levels because of a severe cholesterol problem, reduce intake of foods from animal sources, such as meat (not more than six ounces), poultry, fish, seafood's, and use fat-free or low fat dairy products. High-quality proteins from vegetable sources, like beans, and lentils are excellent substitutes for animal proteins.

Thus, clearly in most cases high cholesterol can be treated with dietary changes and exercise alone. However, to be on the safe side we have discussed specific nutrients (natural supplements) that will help to significantly reduce the cholesterol level without any side effects. Traditional treatment with statin drugs (i.e., Lovastatin, Pravastatin, fluvastatin, atorvastatin) produce serious side effects, including nutritional deficiency, and liver toxicity which may eventually damage the liver. These topics are discussed in detail in later sections.

Thus, clearly in most cases high cholesterol can be treated with dietary changes and exercise alone. However, to be on the safe side we have discussed specific nutrients (natural supplements) that will help to significantly reduce the cholesterol level without any side effects. Conventional treatment with statin drugs (i.e., Lovastatin, Pravastatin, fluvastatin, atorvastatin) produce serious side effects, including nutritional deficiency, and liver toxicity which may eventually damage the liver. These topics are discussed in detail in later sections.

In some cases, doctors may find it necessary to prescribe cholesterol-lowering medications, especially to those patients who are unwilling to make life-style changes or have severe cholesterol problems. If you are concerned about serious side effects and your doctor wants to prescribe cholesterol-lowering medications, you may explain to him that you are willing to start on a regimen that may help avoid the life-long dependency on prescription drugs. Whatever you decide, it must be based on your analysis of your personal conditions.

What Your Cholesterol Levels Mean?

Blood cholesterol levels fall into one of the following categories.

Desirable Level: Less than 200 mg/dl

Border Line High Risk: 200—239 mg/dl

High Risk: 240 mg/dl and over

Below we explain pros and cons of each one of these categories.

Desirable Cholesterol Level

If your cholesterol level is less than 200 mg/dl, risk of heart attack is relatively low, of course barring other complications and/or risk factors. Even with a low cholesterol level, it is still advisable to consume foods low in saturated fats, trans fats, and cholesterol. and get plenty of regular exercise. If you are over 45, get your regular physical check up (it always includes cholesterol levels; LDL, HDL, and triglycerides) at least every two years. However, if you have problems, have checkups frequently

Borderline High Risk Level

People with cholesterol levels from 200 to 239 are considered borderline high risk. Study reports that about one third of American adults are in the borderline group, and nearly half of adults have total cholesterol levels below 200 mg/dl.

You should check/recheck your cholesterol and HDL in one to two years if:

- your total cholesterol is in this range
- your HDL is less than 40 mg/dl
- you don't have other risk factors for heart disease
-

In this situation, you should reduce the intake of foods high in cholesterol, saturated fats, trans fats, and hydrogenated fats to lower blood cholesterol level to below 200 mg/dl. If possible, ask your doctor to get a blood test not only to measure blood cholesterol level, but to get a complete cholesterol analysis, including LDL, HDL levels, ratios LDL/HDL, triglyceride level/HDL level, and apoB/apoA1.

Ask your doctor to explain the results of the analysis to you. Even though one has a total cholesterol level between 200 to 239 mg/dl, it does not necessarily mean that he or she is at high risk for a heart attack. Everyone's case is different. For instance, pre-menopausal women and young active adults without any risk factors—may have high HDL cholesterol and desirable LDL levels

High Risk Cholesterol Level

If your blood cholesterol level is 240 mg/dl or more, you are undoubtedly at higher risk of having a heart attack and/or stroke. Normally, people who have a total blood cholesterol level of 240 mg/dl have twice the risk of coronary heart disease compared to people whose cholesterol level is 199 mg/dl or lower. If you land in this situation, it is advisable to have more detailed tests, and seek your doctor's advice.

Your LDL Cholesterol Level

Your LDL cholesterol level greatly impacts on your risk of coronary diseases, such as heart attack and stroke. The lower your LDL cholesterol level, the lower your risk of coronary diseases. It is a better predictor of risk than total blood cholesterol. Your LDL cholesterol level can be classified as follows:

LDL Cholesterol Level

Less than 100 mg/dl	Optimal
100 to 129 mg/dl	Near Optimal/Above Optimal

130 to 159 mg/dl	Borderline High
160 to 189 mg/dl	High
190 mg/dl and above	Very High

Remember that the lower the LDL level, the lower the risk. With this in mind, if you have cholesterol problems, you must take proper measures to reduce your LDL level, such as regular physical activity, low cholesterol diets, eliminate bad fats (1.e in saturated fats, trans fats, hydrogenated fats, etc) from your daily diets, take antioxidant nutrients. If this does not help and your condition is too severe, then consult your family physician who might prescribe some cholesterol lowering drugs. See later for details.

LDL Level at Which One should Consider Drug Therapy

	Existing LDL Level	Desired Level
People without coronary heart disease and with fewer than two risk factors	190 mg/dl or higher	160 mg/dl or lower
People without coronary heart disease and with two or more risk factors	160 mg/dl or higher	130 mg/dl or lower
People with coronary heart disease	130 mg/dl or higher	100 mg/dl or lower

In any case, you should discuss your problem with health care practitioners if you have one of the above conditions. If you don't know whether you have other risk factors for heart disease check the American Heart Association's list or talk to your doctor.

Your HDL Cholesterol Level

Average HDL level in men ranges from 40 to 50 mg/dl, and in women it ranges from 50 to 60 mg/dl. HDL cholesterol level that is less than 40 mg/dl is considered low. People with a low HDL cholesterol level are at high risk of heart disease

There are several factors that are responsible for a low HDL cholesterol level, for instance smoking, over weight, improper diet. If you have a low HDL level, take note of the following:

- don't smoke
- maintain an ideal health
- have regular activities (30-60 min) every day
- consume healthy foods
- take natural supplements
- stop taking drugs if possible. Drug depletes beneficial nutrients making the body defenseless against a host of diseases

- proper rest, reduce stress
- lower your triglyceride levels. High triglyceride levels affect HDL level

- high blood triglyceride level and lower HDL cholesterol level

  increase the risk of heart attack and stroke

- progesterone, anabolic steroid and male sex hormone (testosterone)

  reduce the HDL level, whereas female sex hormones raise HDL levels

Cholesterol Ratio

Although, the measurement of total blood cholesterol level is the most common practice employed to determine your risk of coronary diseases, there is also another critical step which is equally important is the measurement of HDL or "good" cholesterol level.

However, some physicians prefer to use the ratio of total cholesterol to HDL cholesterol in place of the total blood cholesterol. To obtain the ratio, divide the total cholesterol level by the HDL level. For example, the ratio of a total cholesterol level of 250 mg/dl and HDL cholesterol level of 50 mg/dl is 250/50 = 5:1. One must endeavor to keep the ratio below 5:1; the optimum ratio is 3.5:1.

However, the American Heart Association recommends that the absolute numbers for total blood cholesterol and HDL cholesterol levels be used. The physicians find this more useful than the cholesterol ratio in determining the appropriate treatment for patients.

Cholesterol in Women

Women typically have higher HDL ("good") cholesterol level than men. This is due to the fact that the female sex hormone estrogen tends to elevate the HDL cholesterol level. This explains why pre-menopausal women are normally protected from the risk of developing heart disease. Moreover, estrogen production is highest during child bearing years. Generally, women tend to have higher triglyceride levels. Triglyceride levels range between 60 to 250 mg/dl depending on sex and age. People who are overweight and/or older tend to have elevated triglyceride levels.

Cholesterol in Children

There is strong evidence that the atherosclerotic process (fatty plaque buildups in arteries) begins in childhood and keeps progressing slowly into adulthood. This condition often leads to cardiovascular diseases, the leading cause of death in North America. Although, significant progress has been achieved in the area of reducing deaths due to coronary heart disease over the past decades, this disease is still the leading cause of deaths in North America.

Cholesterol Levels in Children and adolescents 2-19 Years Olds

Desirable ----less than 170 mg/dl

Borderline – 170-199 mg/dl

High -----------200 mg/dl and above

Studies Show That:

- atherosclerosis or its precursors begin early in life
- plaque buildups due to elevated cholesterol early in life may be factors for the development of adult atherosclerosis
- improper diet and genetics may contribute to high blood cholesterol levels and arterial diseases
- lowering cholesterol levels in children and adolescents may be extremely beneficial
- smoking must be discouraged
- increased physical activities should be encouraged
- if your children are overweight, take steps to normalize their weight
- diabetes Type 2 should be diagnosed and treated

Lipid Peroxidation

In order to explain lipid peroxidation or oxidation of cholesterol and how to prevent it we need to introduce important concepts: free radicals and antioxidants.

CHAPTER FIVE

FREE RADICALS AND OXYDATIO OF CHOLESTEROL

Free Radicals

Free radicals or reactive oxygen species are atoms or molecules that contain one or more unpaired electrons, and therefore unstable and highly reactive. Free radicals are lethal or deadly. Strangely enough they are both friend and enemy. They are a part of the normal metabolism of the human body. Since they are highly unstable molecules, they haunt healthy molecules to steal their electros to make them stable. Once they oxidize a healthy molecule, it becomes a new free radical, thereby producing a cascade of free radicals, and causing lethal damage to the body.

As a result, this process unless kept on check will result what we call a free radical cascade, an enormous chain reaction of free radicals that wreaks havoc on the body. This will cause irreparable damage to the body leading to a myriad of chronic degenerative diseases, such as atherosclerosis, stroke, Alzheimer's, Parkinson's, and premature aging. In fact, free radicals may play a major role in the development of heart diseases, strokes, arthritis and other chronic debilitating diseases, primarily by oxidizing polyunsaturated fatty acids in lipoproteins, especially low density lipoproteins (LDL).

You will be surprise to know the magnitude of of the process of oxidation taking place in our body at each moment. Our body contains on average (depending on size) more than 67.2 to 100 trillion cells. During our normal activities (i.e., talking, walking, exercise, having sex, thinking....etc.), each cell produces millions of free radicals. Imagine the flood of free radicals being produced at each moment in your body. If the body has no defense mechanisms against the deluge of free radical production, it will be overwhelmed by them be decrepit and eventually perish.

Fortunately, the body has certain defense mechanisms which consist of a complex antioxidant defense system that eliminate these free radicals. Each time a cell produces free radicals, it also simultaneously produces antioxidants to eliminate them. This continuous battle goes on twenty four hours a day inside our body. The trouble arises if our body is not healthy enough or deficient in beneficial nutrients to produce sufficient antioxidants to win the deadly battle against free radicals, then the body will wilt and prematurely die.

The trouble is that as we get older our antioxidant defense mechanism against free radicals decreases, then they run rampant causing all sorts of damage to the body. This is why we must take diet rich antioxidants and/or antioxidant supplements to keep our body in peak form to win the lethal battle against free radicals. We will talk about antioxidants later. Now having discussed the notions of free radicals and antioxidants, we are ready to discuss oxidation of cholesterol and its effects on the body.

Cholesterol is not the Villain. It is the Oxidation of Cholesterol

There exists no correlation between lowering cholesterol levels and increased longevity. As a matter of fact, the majority of people who get heart attacks or strokes don't have high cholesterol. There are scandalous lies and misguided propaganda against cholesterol. One must understand the serious side effects of artificially lowering cholesterol with cholesterol- lowering drugs and cholesterol artifacts without implementing other beneficial strategies which are critical to maintaining good health.

Framingham Heart Study conducted over five decades proved without doubt that the LDL cholesterol level is just one of many misleading factors of heart disease. Indeed, LDL cholesterol levels are only a trifling factor of heart disease and only on certain conditions. Here is a quote from Christie Ballantyne, M.D., a cardiologist, Bayer College of Medicine "The majority of people who end up having heart attacks or strokes don't have high cholesterol

As a matter of fact, scientific research studies suggest that as people lower their LDL cholesterol, their chances of getting strokes go up. Artificially lowering cholesterol levels by using cholesterol-lowering drugs may increase your risk of death from stroke and heart attack. Furthermore, the increased toxicity due to cholesterol- lowering-drugs could lead to liver and kidney failure. Cholesterol is certainly not unhealthy as has been perceived by the pharmaceutical and medical communities. The conspiracy against cholesterol is due to the enormous financial benefits reaped by the greedy drug pharmaceutical industries by pushing cholesterol-lowering-drugs and cholesterol artifacts. These are more toxic and harmful to health than cholesterol itself.

As we have said before, cholesterol is absolutely essential for the body without which the body may perish. It is required for multitude of bodily functions. Cholesterol is an integral part of each and every cell membrane. It provides the critical starting point and building block for the steroid hormones including sex hormones, such as testosterone, and estrogen. Cholesterol products, such as progesterone, estradiol and testosterone increase serotonin-receptors which make you happy. Moreover, 20 % of the brain is composed of cholesterol, and it is nrain's powerful antioxidant..

Thus, an adequate level of cholesterol is essential for maintaining good health. If your cholesterol level is too low, you will get ill sooner. Low cholesterol level is bad for the brain and liver. If the cholesterol level is too low, it might lead to depression, aggressiveness, and tendency to commit suicide. Indeed, numerous scientific studies have shown that people with a low cholesterol level have attempted or succeeded in committing suicide. The real *culprit* here is the oxidation of cholesterol.

Cholesterol Oxidation: health hazards and antioxidants to rescue

As it is clear from above that cholesterol itself is not too bad. It is the oxidation of cholesterol by free radicals that creates havoc. Free radicals may play a major role in the development of atherosclerosis, stroke, and other degenerative diseases by oxidizing polyunsaturated fatty acids in lipoproteins, especially low-density-lipoproteins (LDL). When cholesterol is oxidized, it becomes "sticky" and start to form plaque in the walls of the arteries, eventually clogging the arteries. This condition obviously makes the arteries narrow, thereby creating blockage in the arteries supplying blood to the heart and brain, eventually leading to heart attack and stroke.

Here is what happens. The cholesterol molecule having a double bond in its structure is more readily susceptible to oxidation forming cholesterol like molecules called oxy-sterols. These harmful oxidized products are found in many of the foods we eat, and which are normally formed during their manufacture and/or processing. The potential toxic effects of oxy-sterol consumption may be highly carcinogenic. The primary dietary sources of oxy-sterols are: eggs and egg-derived products, milk and milk-derived products, foods fried in vegetable/animal oil (French fried potatoes), and also cholesterol containing foods that have been heated and preheated and/or frozen a number of times. These are the main sources of oxy-sterols in the North American diet.

To explain oxidation: just watch an apple turn brown when it is cut open and exposed to air. This is oxidation. Our body will get oxidized on the inside by free radicals unless proper steps are taken to prevent this and also to prevent cholesterol oxidation. This is where antioxidants come to the rescue. The antioxidants not only prevent the oxidation of triglycerides and cholesterols, but also neutralize the free radicals that would have otherwise inflicted the body with a host of degenerative diseases, such as heart attack, stroke, Parkinson's, Alzheimer's, premature aging and death.

Some of the antioxidants that can keep harmful free radicals from damaging cholesterol and the cells of the body are vitamins A, B's, C, E, D, and CoQ10, PQQ, R+-alpha lipoic acid, flavonoid quercetin, pycnogenol, glutathione (marker of life), and also omega-3 fatty acids, fish oil, astaxanthin, and so on. Here is a partial list of a rich source of antioxidant foods: garlic, onion, ginger, olive oil, coconut oil, avocados oil, avocado, eggplants, okras, asparagus, spinach, green beans, broccoli, cabbage, cauliflower, almonds, walnuts, Brazil nuts, pistachio, pumpkin seeds, and fresh fruits, such as apples, kiwi, mangos, grapes, all berries, and cherries

If you are someone who needs help to lower your cholesterol level, read on. There are natural supplements discussed in later sections which will help you lower your cholesterol levels without any side effects. However, we advise you to consult with your healthcare professional before self-treating yourself

CHAPTER SIX

Cholesterol Is Not Your Enmey

Most people are told cardiovascular diseases are due to cholesterol clumping together to form build ups that block the flow of blood.

Cholesterol is a **vital nutrient** your body uses to repair rips, tears, or growths in the walls of your blood vessels. When damage occurs, cholesterol flowing in the blood stops to coat and repair the damaged area. As more layers of cholesterol are added for healing, a bulge of cholesterol is formed. Imagine what will happen to your blood vessels if cholesterol does not repair the rips, tears and growths in the walls of your blood vessels.

 *Unfortunately, these **bulges** are what have given cholesterol its bad reputation.*

Real Cause of Circulation Problems

Research study shows that these healing bulges are not the real cause of heart and circulatory problems.

Your blood vessels are specially made to work around these soft and pliable bulges. Normal arteries simply stretch and increase their diameter around the bulges to let blood flowing normally.

But shocking new research has identified calcium as the major problem in cardiovascular disease. Research studies report that your body is not very efficient to properly utilize calcium. In fact, only about one fourth of calcium you take is being absorbed in a form usable to your bones, teeth, muscles. The remaining 75 % floats around your body until it is eliminated as waste.

Unfortunately, before it can be eliminated, a lot of these unusable calcium gets deposited in your tissues and joints causing wrinkles and arthritis.

The most deadly problem is: Calcium Hardens Your Arteries

The cholesterol bulges are the favorite dumping ground for unused calcium. Instead of staying soft and pliable, the bulge fills with calcium and becomes a hardened (calcified) rock called plaque

Moreover, when the bulge hardens, the entire artery wall becomes inflexible with atherosclerosis leading to serious health problems like high blood pressure, fatigue, breathlessness, chest pain, heart attacks...

What is worst, because of the lack of flexibility, your blood vessels can no longer expand. Hence any pieces of clotted blood could block your arteries causing heart attack or debilitating or deadly stroke.

Reference: Dr. Richard Cohen, M>D., Health Research Labs

Why Then Are There So Many Scandalous Lies about Cholesterol?

There are billions of dollars being made at the expense of people's health by selling cholesterol-level-lowering drugs and cholesterol artifacts (i.e., margarine, vegetable shortening, and artificial egg products). This deceit becomes even more malicious knowing that the cholesterol-lowering drugs can cause severe side-effects, such as pancreas cancer, liver tumors, kidney failures, cancer, and cognitive dementia. As we have mentioned before, if the cholesterol level becomes too low, then it might lead to depression, aggression, and inclination to commit suicide and murder. Consult the following reference for other dangerous side effects of statin drugs.

Ref: STATIN DANGERS: Cholesterol Lowering Drugs, such as lipitor, Zicor......induce

heart failure and more......; by *Sally Fallon and Mary G. Enig, Ph.D.*

Kevin Trudeau, **The Natural Cures "They" Don't Want You To Know About**

Symptoms

Typically high cholesterol symptoms can be totally undetectable. Indeed, most people don't feel any high cholesterol symptoms, and only to find out later when they get coronary disease and stroke. Even though you don't see any high cholesterol symptoms, it does not mean that you don't have high cholesterol levels. In any case it is advisable to ask your doctor to check your cholesterol levels at regular intervals, say every one or two years. Moreover, in case the following situations apply to you, there is a high degree of possibility that your cholesterol levels are high:

- you eat fast and fried foods
- regularly eat diary and diary products
- regularly eat processed foods, including deli products
- indulge in fatty meats—ribs, bacon, sausage, beef and/or pork chops
- sedentary life style
- regular smoker
- if you are overweight, your body stores fats and cholesterol

In this case and in the absence of high cholesterol symptoms, you need to check your blood cholesterol levels frequently, at least once in every year or even every six month.

Although, high cholesterol symptoms are not detectable, you can actually observe them from the end results of high cholesterol, such as heart attack and stroke. One indication of high cholesterol can be a buildup of cholesterol rings on the skin under the eyes. Look for symptoms as described below:

- dizziness, loss of balance
- mental confusion or dullness
- circulatory problems, sweating
- difficulty in breathing after minor exertion or shortness of breath

Since high cholesterol symptoms are silent, it is imperative that you check your cholesterol levels with your doctor, and ask him to explain the numbers to you.

Root Causes

Several factors can affect your blood cholesterol levels. Some of these factors you can control and others you can't.

You can control

- you can control what you eat. Certain foods and fats raise your cholesterol levels.

saturated fats raise your low density lipoprotein (LDL) cholesterol levels more

than anything else in your diet.

trans fats (trans fatty acids) are made when vegetable oils are hydrogenated to

harden. Trans fatty acids raise cholesterol levels

cholesterol found in foods from animal sources, such as egg yolks, meat and

meat products, diary and dairy products

- **overweight**. Being overweight may lead to increase in LDL)bad) cholesterol levels, lowers your HDL (good) cholesterol levels, and increases your total cholesterol levels
- **sedentary life style.** Lack of regular exercise may lead to weight gain, which in turn raises your cholesterol levels. Regular exercise can help you lose weight; thereby helping you lower yours LDL cholesterol level and raise your HDL cholesterol levels.
- Diabetes, insulin resistance
- Hypothyroidism
- Stress

You can't control

- **Heredity:** a certain inherited genetic condition, such as familial hypercholesterolemia can result in very high LDL cholesterol levels. This begins at birth and may lead to a heart attack at an early age.
- **Age and Sex:** starting at puberty, men have lower HDL cholesterol levels than women. But LDL cholesterol levels rise in both men and women as they get older. Although younger women have lower LDL cholesterol levels than men, however, after age 55 women have higher levels than men.

Testing Procedures

Total cholesterol, HDL, LDL, VLDL, apoB, apoA-1, triglyceride levels---all are blood tests

Oxidative damage---blood or urine

CHAPTER SEVEN

FIBER AND FOODS CAN HELP LOWER CHOLESTEROL

Health Benefits of Fiber

Fibre , a less trendy term is "roughage." Traditionally, fibre was considered to be an inert part of food, passing undigested from mouth to anus and excreted intact in the stool. Our modern diets contain hardly any fibre, which in turn lead to constipation, diverticular, high blood cholesterol, obesity, diabetes, heart disease, stroke and cancer.

There are two types of fibers, "**soluble and insoluble**."

Insoluble Fiber

Its job is to make stools heavier and speed their passage thru the gut. It functions like a sponge that can absorb many times its weight in water, swelling up and help eliminate feces and allay constipation. Some of the rich sources of insoluble fibre are: wheat bran, barley, couscous, brown rice, bulgur, wheat bran, as well as the skins of many fruits and vegetables, nuts and seeds.

As the outer fibre layer is often removed by food processing due to milling, pealing, boiling or extracting, thus, it is advisable to eat unrefined foods to get insoluble fibre.

Insoluble Fiber

Its job is to make stools heavier and speed their passage thru the gut. It functions like a sponge that can absorb many times its weight in water, swelling up and help eliminate feces and allay constipation. Some of the rich sources of insoluble fibre are: wheat bran, barley, couscous, brown rice, bulgur, wheat bran, as well as the skins of many fruits and vegetables, nuts and seeds.

As the outer fibre layer is often removed by food processing due to milling, pealing, boiling or extracting, it is advisable to eat unrefined foods to get insoluble fibre.

Soluble Fiber

This type of fibre is found in foods which includes pectin (such as apples), guar gum, betaglucans, oats, legumes (peas, beans, lentils), brown rice, barley, fruits (apples, pears, berries, prunes, kiwi), green vegetables (i.e., broccoli, green beans, Brussels sprout, spinach, mustard greens, zucchini, cauliflower..), and potatoes. Soluble fibre breaks down; it passes through the digestive tract forming a gel that traps some harmful substances concerning cholesterol. Soluble fibre absorbs fat. Cholesterol being a fat, it absorbs cholesterol, thereby helping to reduce high cholesterol levels.

Study shows that people who consume a high fibre diet have lower total cholesterol levels and may be less likely to form dangerous blood clots than those who consume less soluble fibre. Several studies showed that sufficient consumption of fibre in our diet apparently can reduce total blood cholesterol level, heart disease, as well as allay diverticular disease, hemorrhoids, bowel cancer, diabetes and insulin resistance, and regulate blood sugar level as well.

Soluble fibre increases the excretion of bile acids from the body through the colon. When these acids are excreted, more cholesterol is used by the liver to replace them. This means that the more acids are made, the more cholesterol is drawn out of the body, and hence there is less risk of cholesterol being deposited in the arteries which cause blood pressure, heart disease, and strokes.

short chain fatty acids

We will briefly mention how **short chain fatty acids** are formed and their significant

health benefits.

Soluble fibre undergoes active fermentation by the action of colonic bacteria on the food mass producing short chain fatty acids--*butyric, ethanoic, propionic*, and *valeric* acids-- that have significant health benefits, especially butyric acid. See below:

- regulates blood glucose levels by stimulating pancreatic insulin release and liver   control of glycogen breakdown
- keeps a check on cholesterol synthesis by the liver and reduce LDL cholesterol levels and triglyceride levels responsible for heart ailments
- reduces colonic pH (i.e. increase in the acidity levels in the colon) which protects the inner lining of colon from cancer polyp formation and improves absorption of minerals.
- activates production of T-helper cells, antibodies, leukocytes, cytokines, and lymph mechanism exerting critical role in immune protection
- boosts proliferation of colonic bacteria—bifidobacteria and lactobacilli, for intestinal health;
- deters colonic inflammation and adhesion irritants.

In summary, fermentable fibres produce the beneficial short-chain fatty acids that affect blood glucose and lipid levels, fortify colonic environment and regulate immune responses.

Tips for adding more Fibre to Your Diet

- start with a nutritious breakfast that includes oats, or a serving of high-fibre cereal (e.g., all-bran Kellog's cereal or bran flakes), raisins with milk, an apple or strawberry, blueberries or a fruit of your choice. You may add Chia seeds or sprinkle some psyllium if possible.
- Try brown rice
- Consume fruits like apples, peaches, prunes, grapes, pears, and dried fruits like raisins (raisin has sugar, should not use), cranberries, all berries, prunes, dates and apricots
- Eat more unpeeled and well washed fresh fruits and vegetables, lentils, beans
- Another way to enrich fibre content in your diet is to supplement it with fibre, guar gum, psyllium, or pectin (apples)

Inulin

Inulin is a natural soluble fibre made from chicory root. It is a long chain dietary fibre found in over 36,000 edible plant species. It is also present in many common fruits and vegetables, such as artichokes, asparagus, leeks, onions, garlic, resins, and bananas. Higher concentrations exist in herbs, such as Dandelion roots, elecampane root and chicory root all have large amounts of inulin.

Health Benefits Of Inulin

- **Inulin** help increase growth of friendly bacteria in your gut that fortify the body's the body's natural defenses, preventing common digestive ailments and thus promoting digestive health
- **inulin** may lower blood triglycerises and cholesterol
- **Inulin** may lower risk of diabetes
- **Inulin** promotes weight loss
- **Bone Health:** Linulin improves absorption of calcium and magnesium leading to improved bone density in adolescents and postmenopausal women
- **Colon Cancer:** research showed that inulin may reduce precancerous colon growth and support a less favorable environment for colon cancer development in humans
- **Constipation:** daily supplements of 15 grams (try smaller dose first) of inulin improved constipation and quality of life in elderly people with constipation
- **Inulin** can add nutritional value to foods while improving taste and texture. It dissolves completely in virtually any liquid (hot or cold) and in soft foods as well without altering flavor and texture.
- **Caution:** women who are pregnant and/or breastfeeding avoid use of inuin

Oats vs Oat Bran, and Heart Disease

For last thirty years there are over twenty major studies have been conducted to examine the relationships concerning oats, oat bran, and cholesterol levels. An individual whose cholesterol level is over 200 mg/dl, a bowl of oats or oat bran may mean a great deal to his health. In fact, daily intake of such a bowl could lower his risk of heart disease by 50 %. It is known that a bowl of oatmeal has about three grams of fibre, and it is these three grams of water-soluble oat fibre that can lower cholesterol level nearly 8 to 23 percent.

Moreover, every 1 percent drop in cholesterol levels can help reduce the risk of heart disease by 2 percent. The daily intake of a bowl of oatmeal lowers one's risk of heart disease by between 16 and 46 percent. However, this does not affect people with normal or low cholesterol levels with daily consumption of oats, which will produce little or no change in cholesterol levels.

IN CLOSING

Try to eat your last meal of the day no later than 7:30 PM. This will, especially solve common and serious problems with diabetes and/or obese people: eating—and overeating—at night, especially a big meal two hours before bed time will lead to impairment of the digestive systems, and/or obesity; it will cause blood flow to the stomach not to the brain.. At night most of us have time to sit down for a big meal. Clinical studies have shown that most overweight people with diabetes eat more calories at night than at any other time of the day. However, this large amount of calories is exactly the opposite of what people with diabetes and obesity need.

At night our metabolism winds down as our body prepares for sleep. Thus, intake of calories at night are more likely to be stored as fat, making you more obese which could lead to various degenerative diseases, such as high serum cholesterol levels, heart disease, strokes, diabetes, and cancer. Moreover, eating this late in the day makes the body work harder for digestion, thus obstructing the important process of tissue repairs and muscle building, and other rejuvenating work that is being carried out by the body during restful sleep

Therefore, eating heavy meals just before bed time not only obstruct the important processes of repairs and rejuvenation, but also lead to impairment of the digestive system and make the blood flow to the stomach instead of the brain which could cause brain disorders. Make sure to eat your heavy meal at least four hours before bed time.

Diabetes

Soluble fiber in oat bran, oatmeal, legumes (dried beans of all kinds, peas, lentils), and pectin (from fruits, such as apples) is considered, especially beneficial for people with diabetes type 2 or type 1. Since the fiber slows down the digestion of foods (especially, carbohydrates), thereby helping blunt the sudden spikes in blood glucose that generally occurs after a low-fiber meal. Such blood glucose spikes stimulate the pancreas to pump more insulin whose accumulative effect over the years may contribute to diabetes type 2, which typically strikes after the age of 40, and more than doubles the risk of heart disease and strokes. However, the cholesterol lowering activity of soluble fiber may help those diabetes sufferers with reduced risk of heart disease and strokes.

Blood sugar problems, such as hypoglycemia, insulin resistance, diabetes and Alzheimer (now considered as type 3 diabetes) are closely linked to diets lacking in fiber. Fiber helps in improving glucose tolerance. Several clinical studies have shown that supplementing diets with fiber have proven to show beneficial effects in improving blood sugar control. High fiber diets help prevent diabetes type 2, and also improve blood sugar control for people with diabetes. People with higher cereal fiber consumption are 64 % less likely to develop diabetes.

Some of the best fiber sources to consume for weight loss are psyllium, guar gum, gum karaya, and pectin (apples), since they are rich in water-soluble fibre. Drink a lot of water.

Caution: if you have a disorder in the esophagus, do not take fiber supplement in pill form. They may expand in the esophagus causing serious problem.

Ideally, healthy adults should consume 26 to 35 grams of fiber daily. The present average consumption by North Americans is somewhere between 4.5 to 11 grams a day. Health Canada recommends an increase in this amount by taking more grains (may be diabetes should not take grains, since they are rapidly metabolized thereby increasing in blood glucose spikes), unpeeled and properly washed fruits and vegetables. Include both soluble and insoluble fiber in your diet. Furthermore, a fibre-rich diet provides plenty of vitamins and minerals.

For Prediabetes, Diabetes, or blood sugar problems: Take cinnamon (sprinkle on your food, add to your soup or tea) and chromium picolinate, 200 mcg twice daily.

CHAPTER EIGHT

Treatments to Lower Cholesterol Levels

DIET

- Modern American diets are one of the causes of high cholesterol. For instance, fried foods, processed foods, processed meats, trans fats, saturated fats. There is no way you will be healthy if you are eating regularily foods that are being offered in fast food chains.
  Take oatmeal and oat bran in your breakfast. They have been known to reduce cholesterol levels It is clear from the above discussions that the major key to balancing cholesterol levels is to consume fibre-rich diets. This means go overboard with fruits and vegetables in your diet, also take nuts and seeds as snacks.
  one bowl of oatmeal daily can reduce cholesterol levels between 8 to 23 percent in just three weeks.
  Remember every 1 percent drop in cholesterol level brings the risk of heart disease down 2 percent, and a daily intake of a bowl of oatmeal lowers the risk by between 16 and 46 percent.
- If you just eliminate processed foods, fried foods and bad fats from your diet, including refined sugar and carbohydrates, your cholesterol level will be substantially reduced. People with diabetes can dramatically reduce their cholesterol level if they adopt the suggestions given above and increase their consumption of complex carbohydrates and protein, especially vegetable proteins, such as beans, of all kinds and lentils.

  Take avocado everyday. It has numerous health benefits, including lowering cholesterol level, weight loss, and heart health.

Foods Recommended

Taking soluble fibre in your diet will not only dramatically lower cholesterol levels, but also reduce the risk of various other diseases, such as heart disease, stroke, diabetes, diverticular disease, colon cancer. The rich sources of this fiber can be found in oats, brown rice, whole wheat (don't take wheat or wheat products), beans, lentils, fruits and vegetables. For breakfast take a bowl of hot oatmeal, flavored with milk (soy? No), raisins, strawberries, or bananas and a little blackstrap molasses or raw honey. Take also an apple, orange, or a pear on the side.

The molecules in cholesterol are extremely susceptible to oxidative damage by highly reactive oxygen species (known as free radicals). This is generally known as lipid peroxidation, which could lead to heart disease and other serious chronic ailments. In order to prevent oxidation of cholesterol, one must take antioxidant-rich fruits and vegetables, especially deeply colored fruits and vegetables. Consume wide varieties of fruits and vegetables for the broad-ranging protection, and eat at least five or six lightly cooked (raw if possible) servings of vegetables daily. Take avocado every day. It has many health benefits, including heart health, reducing high cholesterol level and weight loss.

Avocado is perhaps the best overall source of glutathione, the master antioxidant.

It's Levels in the blood indicates how long a person is going to live.. Ounce-per-ounce it ranks highest in essential fatty acids, monounsaturated fats, vitamin E, foliate, potassium, magnesium, lutein, beta-sitosterol. It is considered as one of the supper guardians of cells because of its abundance of glutathione, the "master anti-oxidant" that effectively neutralize highly lethal destructive fats in food. Although, avocado is high in fat, much of it is good fat monounsaturated, a type of fat that resist oxidation. It is also helpful in reducing high blood pressure, since it is a rich source of potassium.

According to recent research, avocado can lower blood cholesterol levels and increase HDL cholesterol levels, because it contain oleic acid, a monoun-saturated fat that helps lower total cholesterol. Studies have shown that people on diet that include avocado for seven days showed significant decrease in total blood cholesterol and LDL cholesterol, along with an 11 % increase in health promoting HDL cholesterol. Avocados, contain high quantities of monounsaturated fatty acids, including oleic acids, which has recently been shown to lend significant protection against breast cancer as well as prostate cancer. It also contains all the carotenoid families (lutein, alpha-carotene, beta-carotene, zeaxanthin) and significant amounts of vitamin E.

According to "Wilen Sisters", avocado could really lower your cholesterol upto 42 %. Avocado is not only packed with heart-healthy omega-9 fatty acids, but is also rich in the compound called beta-sitosterol which has been known to lower cholesterol in 16 different studies.

A research study at Ohio State University reported that avocado acts as a "nutrient-booster" letting the body to substantially improve absorption of heart-healthy and cancer fighting nutrients like alpha-carotene, beta-carotene, zeaxanthin and lycopene found in fruits and vegetables. It even supplies more potassium than banana.

As avocado is easily digested, this makes it an ideal food for people recovering from surgery or who are very sick. Furthermore, consumption of avocado stabilizes blood sugar levels and cleanses the liver. Scientists believe that avocado may be beneficial in the treatment of hepatitis (liver cancer) as well as other sources of liver damages. It is also well known that avocado may help lose weight.

Avocado can heal people with digestive and circulatory conditions.

Traditionally, avocado is reputed to have helped people with sexual problems as well as skin conditions.

Contraindications: don't take avocado if you are taking anti-depressant drug MAOI.

Ref: Schwartz, SJ. *Caretonoid Absorption from Salad and Salsa by Humans is enhanced by the addition of avocado or avocado oil.* J. Nutr. March

Apple: Here are some of the familiar adages:

"to eat an apple going to bed, will make the doctor beg his bread,"

"an apple a day can keep breast cancer away,"

"an apple a day keeps Alzheimer's disease at bay."

"an apple a day keeps a doctor away."

" an apple a day keep cholesterol at bay"

Apple contains powerful antioxidants and has a wide range of health-rich benefits from weight loss to hair retention to type 2 diabetes. If your daily diet includes apples, you will fall ill less frequent

Brazilian researchers chronicled that participants in the research study who ate an apple at every meal lost more weight while dieting than participants who did not eat fruit in their clinical trial.

Finish researchers have documented that people who eat apples have a reduced risk of several degenerative chronic diseases, including heart disease, cancer, strokes, type 2 diabetes, and asthma. This is also confirmed by the research studies conducted at Cornell University which reported that apple consumption promotes hair growth and weight loss, keeps skin from wrinkling, controls blood sugar, anti-aging, prevents bladder cancer, lung cancer, prostate cancer, strokes, heart disease, and helps reduce cholesterol.

A French Study also discovered that the compound **procyanidines** in ordinary apples were extremely effective in killing dangerous cancer cells. Just be sure to the whole apple, because of the many of the cancer-fighting nutrients are found in the apple's skin.

Apples are a rich source of pectin fibre that binds to fats (hence cholesterol) and heavy metals for elimination.

Other health benefits:

* apple cleans teeth and strengthens gum

* detoxifies the system and has an antiviral activity

* helps digestion and prevents constipation

* enriches your diet with fibre

An average apple contains roughly 80 calories, 5 grams of fibre (20 % of daily requirements) and almost no fat or cholesterol. The fibre (pectin) in apple helps to make us feel fuller. This in part is the reason why apple may be helpful in reducing weight.

3-Apple-a-Day-Plan:

suggests that eating an apple before each meal, the complex sweetness of apples helps gratify the sugar cravings (thereby stops the blood sugar spikes to the brain), while the juice keeps the body hydrated, and also means most likely eating less of things you (and your waist line) will regret..

The new research from Cornell University indicated that apples can protect the brain from oxidative damage that triggers neurodegenerative disorders, such as Alzheimer's and Parkinson's

- offer anti-cancer, antioxidant, and cardiovascular benefits
- eating an apple and drinking apple juice today may protect your brain health tomorrow
- apple is an excellent source of pectin fibre and is well known to be effective to reduce cholesterol in liver and serum cholesterol
- eating apples offers protective benefit to the digestive system, colon, lungs, cancer, heart and brain health

Research studies indicate that eating apples and drinking apple juice which possess a unique mix of antioxidants, lead to increased production of the brain chemical acetylcholine resulting in improved cognition and memory. Apples are potent detoxifiers and apple juice can destroy viruses in the body.

According to Riu Hai Liu of Cornell University, although an apple contains a small amount of vitamin C, eating 100 grams of apple provides the same amount of antioxidant activity as taking 1,500 mg of the same vitamin.

There are numerous reasons to enjoy an "apple a day": **keeps your body young.**

Note: Canadian scientists say: Red delicious apples have more antioxidants, namely polyphenols than seven other apple varieties.

Ref:

http://www.3appleplan.com

http://www.whfoods:apples

vitamins deary apple html

Garlic, onion, ginger, turmeric, fenugreek and cayenne are savory complements to any meal (vegetarian or non-vegetarian meals), and they also help reduce LDL cholesterol levels while increasing HDL cholesterol levels.

Adding spices to our meals, such as turmeric, fenugreek powder, cinnamon, cayenne, basil, rosemary, and oregano not only bring savory taste to foods, but also their richness in antioxidants help prevent oxidation of cholesterol.

Snacking on nuts, especially walnuts or almonds, has been known to lower cholesterol and triglyceride levels.

Not all fats are bad. There are good fats and there are bad fats. Essential fatty acids (EFA) is an extremely good fat and it has numerous health benefits, including cholesterol-lowering and heart-protecting effects. Be sure to enrich your diet with EFA, richly available in cold-water fish, such as salmon, mackerel, cod and sardines. Another rich source of EFA is flaxseeds or flax oil (don't take flax product; it becomes toxic once it is in stomach). Actually salba or chia seeds are the richest source of EFA. You can sprinkle chia seeds or salba on salads, cereals, soup and yogurt.

Cholesterol and Fats

As it is clear from above there are good fats and bad fats. Typically North American diets are rich in bad fats, consisting of fatty meats, processed cold cuts, diary products, fried foods, processed foods and margarine. As if these were not enough, add to this the intake of commercially baked breads, roles, cakes, chips and cookies. This is a surefire road to increased high blood cholesterol.

Oddly enough, consuming cholesterol will not increase the blood cholesterol level nearly as much as eating foods loaded with **saturated fats** and **trans fats** (margarine)**.** Like cholesterol, saturated fat is mainly contained in animal products, such as meats, whole milk, cheese, cream, ice cream, butter, and lard.

One might think changing to vegetable oil one can solve the problem. However, one has to be careful what kind of vegetable oil you are using. Some of the vegetable oils have high content of saturated fat, such as palm oil, palm kernel oil (87 %), cocoa butter (62 %), and butter (66 %). Unfortunately, these are some of the oils most often used in commercially available food products, such as baked goods, nondairy whipped toppings, and fried foods Make sure to read the labels what you are eating.

Other vegetable oils that contain moderate amounts of saturated fat are: canola oil (7%), safflower oil (9%), sunflower oil (11%), olive oil (14 %), sesame oil (15 %), peanut oil (18 %). Canola and olive oil are considered two of the best available cooking oils. Olive oil contains a very high amount of monounsaturated fat, 74%, where as canola oil has 58%. Olive oil has numerous health benefits, including heart health.

My advice is not to use canola oil at all. it gets oxidized in high heat causing bad effects on healt. also it is not good for health. Use instead coconut oil which has numerous health benefits, including heart, brain, and memory.

Trans fatty acids (trans fat) are as bad as saturated fat, and also hydrogenated fat. Margarine and some processed foods contain these fats. stay away from these fats. Consume oils low in saturated fats. Do not consume anything containing trans fat.

Foods to Avoid

By eliminating bad fats, such as saturated, hydrogenated, and trans fats, you can lower cholesterol levels and improve your arterial health. Foods that are dangerously full of these bad fats are: fried foods, sweet baked goods, most crackers, processed foods, cold cuts, and animal products. Often doctors advise patients with high cholesterol to use margarine and vegetable shortening as substitutes for butter and lard, however, these items are high in partially hydrogenated fats which are even more lethal to health than the saturated kind.

Eliminate consumption of alcohol and simple carbohydrates (i.e., white flour, white sugar), including sodas, pops, candy, and baked goods, which tend to stimulate liver to produce more cholesterol. Also reduce intake of caffeine (coffee or black tea, a cup or two a day), which has been linked to high cholesterol. Instead use herbal teas, such as green tea, white tea, chamomile which contain antioxidants that can prevent cholesterol oxidation.

Note: Recent news reported by CTV: research studies indicate that one pop a day increases the risk of heart disease by 44 %. Furthermore new study shows that, one pop a day will reduce your lifespan by 4.6 years. Now imagine the combined effects of health hazards that is being created by consuming pops, trans fats, saturated fats, fried foods, processed foods and others.

- **spreads,** margarine is loaded with trans fat and saturated fats, both of them can lead to heart disease. Moreover, other non- butter spreads and shortenings also have high contents of trans fat and saturated fat.
- **packaged goods,** cake mixes, bisquick, and other mixes all have large amounts of trans fat per serving.
- **soups,** ramen noodles and soup cups have very high levels of trans fat.
- **fast Foods,** really bad news here: fried chicken, French fries, and other foods are deep fried in partially hydrogenated oil, and fries are sometimes partially fried in trans fat prior to their shipping to the restaurant. Pancakes and grilled sandwiches also have some fat.
- **frozen foods,** the tasty frozen pies, pot pies, waffles, pizzas, and breaded fish sticks, all contain trans fat. Even vegetable pizzas are not flawless. The pizza dough likely to contain trans fat. Pot pies are loaded with saturated fat.
- **baked goods,** they are even worse. All commercially baked goods use more trans fat than any other foods. Now we list a few of them without any discussion, such as chips, crackers, cookies, cereals (Kellogg'sCracklin' Oat), chocolate cookies, toppings and dips.

Butter vs Margarine

The high level of saturated fats in butter puts this animal food in the same "don't" class with meats by many. Butter is actually a healthy food with lots of benefits. Eating butter can protect you from skin cancer.

Unfortunately, margarine, touted as the chosen alternative to butter, on the other hand, is more dangerous than smoking cigarettes. The trans fatty acids in it are poison to your arteries leading to hardening of the arteries, yet many people are still brain washed to believe that margarine is good for health. As a matter of fact, margarine is one of the most damaging foods a person can eat. Just try to cut back trans fat if you can't totally eliminate it.

Studies have shown that margarine not only raises the LDL (bad) cholesterol levels, but also reduces the protective HDL (good) cholesterols. Furthermore, it hinders the metabolism of essential fatty acids which are essential for good health. Margarine may cause cancer and hardening of the arteries. Butter also should be restricted in any good diet.

CHAPTER NINE

CHOLESTEROL BEYOND HYPE

Dr. Douglass says and I quote: "Cholesterol is not toxic sludge, but the MOTHER OF ALL NUTRIENTS!"

The purpose of this section is to let you know the report of various studies and the varying degrees of opinions of doctors, especially Dr. William Campbell Douglass II, M.D., relating to the reduction of cholesterol levels, and its effect on health and well-being.

Furthermore, results of the Northern Manhattan Study shows that .

The researchers that conducted the study found that *higher LDL cholesterol was linked to LOWER stroke risk.*[1]

And another study published this year reviewed research on nearly 70,000 people. The authors of that study found *NO LINK between LDL cholesterol and premature deaths in people over 60 from heart disease*.

NowtTo begin the discussions, it has been shown that lowering cholesterol levels won't lower heart attacks. Most people who have heart attacks have normal cholesterol levels. In fact, people with low cholesterol levels will die younger than those with high cholesterol levels.

As we mentioned before, we won't be able to survive without cholesterol. Our body needs cholesterol, and lots of it, steroid hormones (e.g., DHEA, Growth Hormones,), and all sex hormones, such as estrogen, progesterone, and testosterone.

Studies have shown that higher cholesterol could slash your risk of stroke by 300 %.

Here are some of his significant thoughts on cholesterol:

- is your cholesterol high enough to prevent heart disease and strokes?
- one should panic if his or her cholesterol level is less than 200 IU, contrary to conventional medical advise.
- keep your cholesterol level higher than 200 IU
- higher cholesterol is actually one of the greatest health blessings nature has bestowed

Furthermore, higher cholesterol levels can:

- revive and super-charge your sex life
- improve your memory, stave off depression and even protect you from Alzheimer's
- make you far less likely to die

On the other hand, low cholesterol level can:

- actually make arteries harder: you will be surprised to learn that the cholesterol-cutting research studies find that artery clogging was far worse in the patients being treated
- cause massive stroke because of weak blood vessels which have likelihood of being burst open
- likelihood of causing cancer, impair brain function, cause Alzheimer's
- be linked to depression and suicide
- studies have shown that low cholesterol levels can cause cancer

The standard cholesterol test does not give you the true picture of what's really happening with your blood lipids. You should ask your doctor for a VAP test or a lipid subfraction test which will show an expanded lipid profiles that demonstrates what kind of HDL and LDL. This information especially required if you have significant risk factors for heart disease like diabetes, high blood pressure or a family history of heart disorders. This always indicates some degree of inherent risks for heart disease.

The more detail lipid test is available from:

www.spectracell.com

this is an excellent labs.

Beyond Cholesterol, The Three tests

That Could Save Your Life

Cholesterol is a poor indicator of cardiovascular health. The most accurate predictors or marker of cardiovascular health are blood levels of:

- **Triglycerides**
- **Homocysteine**
- **C-reactive protein (CRP)**

Next time you go to your doctor for blood test, ask him for the tests of the three important markers of cardiovascular health.

Triglycerides Levels

Normal is less than 150 mg/dL

High   150 mg/dl to 499 mg/dl

Very high   500 mg/dl or above

Homocysteine

Cholesterol protects your arteries. The real culprit is **homocysteine.** The research studies show that this substance is the real killer, literally eating away your artery walls. Our body repairs by slapping on cholesterol to patch the holes. If it did not, blood vessels in our brain might burst, resulting in massive stroke and death.

Keep your homocysteine levels in check. It is an amino acid that accumulates in our tissues. It is a natural byproduct of cell metabolism. You could consider it as a "waste product." People with high levels of homocysteine are at a greater risk of heart disorders, Alzheimer's, Parkinson's, stroke, and impotence. Diet, genetics, low thyroid, B vitamins and a high animal protein diet increase homocysteine levels.

Your family physician can measure the **homocysteine** levels with a simple blood test.

Normal Range is less than 10 micro mol/L

You can lower your homocysteine levels and keep in check safely and naturally without drugs. For instance, the following list of natural ingredients can not only help lower your homosysteine levels, but also keep it in check. You can find them in any health food stores.

- B12, 500 mcg
- Folic acid, 500 mcg
- Vitamin B6, 25mg
- B2 (Riboflavin), 25 mg

- TMG (Trimethyleine), 500 mg
- *choline* and *trimethylglycine (TMG)*. TMG is also known as *betaine*

If you do some searching, you may find all these ingredients in some or most multi - vitamins.

C-reactive protein is a marker of inflammation in the body, including in the blood vessel walls. It is considered the most accurate predictor of heart disease.

Normal Range is less than 32 mg/dl

The following natural ingredients will lower CRP levels:

- Multivitamin
- Magnesium
- Vitamins E, C and D3
- cholin
- CoQ10, Krill oil
- Omega-3 fatty acids
- Curcumin

Eat more vegetables

Reference:

For more information Consult the book entitled *"Lowering Cholesterol with Nutrition and Natural Supplements, safely"* By **Dr. Art T Dash, M.Sc., M. S., Ph. D. Retired Professor, Published by AuthorHouse, Call 888-519-5121, also advertise in Amazon**

CHAPTER TEN

SERIOUS SIDE EFFECTS OF CHOLESTEROL

LOWERING STATIN DRUGS

Now Decision Time:

Having read **CHOLESTEROL BEYOND HYPE** you may find that you may not need any drug therapy or any other therapeutic treatments depending on your cholesterol level.

Important Suggestion: before you decide to begin treatment either with traditional drug therapy or natural supplements, you should give granulated lecithin a try. It has the reputation of clearing up the cholesterol deposits or bumps even from under the skin.

Dose: take one 1 tbsp twice daily. You may add to juice, soup, or sprinkle on salads, or any thing you are eating.

In case you decide to take lecithin, you probably need a chelated calcium supplement to keep phosphorous and calcium in balance, since choline in lecithin seems to increase the body's phosphorous.

If you have some health conditions or taking prescription drugs, consult with your family physician first before taking lecithin for any drug contraindications.

Now we begin:

Cholesterol Lowering Drugs (Statin drugs)

The following is a list of cholesterol lowering drugs.

- Statins: alorvastatin (Lipitor), Simvastatin (Zocor), Lovastatin (Mevacor), Pravastatin (Pravachol), Rosuvastatin (Crestor), and others

- Bile acid Sequestrants
- Nicotinic Acid
- Fibrates
- Hormone Replacement Therapy

Serious Side Effects of Statin Drugs
Any patient taking these drugs should be regularly monitored by his physician for any serious side effects. These drugs have potentially harmful side effects, such as upset stomach, gas, constipation, abdominal pain or cramps, nausea, diarrhea. Other symptoms are: abnormalities in blood tests of the liver. You may also experience symptoms, such as muscle soreness, joint pain and weakness or brown urine, contact your doctor right away. These drugs eventually may lead to liver damage

Increased blood sugar or risk of type 2 diabetes

Neurological side effects: memory loss or confusion, dementia, cognitive damage

See Jonathan Campbell; Lipitor—Reports of Neuromuscular Degeneration Health Supreme. March 16, 2004

New media explorer sepp 2004 03 18 lipitor side effects and natural remedy htm

Statin Drugs May Increase Risk of Peripheral Neuropathy

Other Side Effects

Sleep problems, sexual function problems, fatigue, dizziness and a sense of detachment are also reported with these drugs. Additionally, people have mentioned experiencing swelling, shortness of breath, vision changes, changes in temperature regulation, weight change, hunger, breast enlargement, blood sugar changes, dry skin, rashes, blood pressure changes, nausea, upset stomach, bleeding, and ringing in ears or other noises.

Note: Recent reports have implicated Lipitor as a possible cause of severe neuromuscular degeneration. Furthermore, people who have been taking Lipitor, sometimes experience symptoms similar to multiple sclerosis (MS), ALS-Lou Gehrig's Disease—in which they lose neuromuscular control of their bodies.

Cholesterol dose not cause heart disease. Countless studies prove beyond doubt that the majority of people who suffer heart attacks have *normal cholesterol levels.* This makes cholesterol-lowering drugs (statins) irrelevant and useless, and *could cost you your life.*

Cholesterol is innocent and misunderstood. The real culprit is inflammation in the arteries, and the drug pushing pharmaceutical industries, not cholesterol. The American Heart Association has discovered that people with heart disease all have one factor in common, and it is not high cholesterol, it is inflammation in their arteries.

What causes inflammation in the arteries? It is *homocysteine,* a harmless acid-like waste product formed when you eat red meat and other protein foods. Homocysteine is rapidly broken down by certain B-complex vitamins. However, if a person lacks B vitamins, which is mostly the case, then homocysteine builds up to dangerous levels and "burns" the delicate tissue of the artery walls.

This leads to plaque formation at the site of this inflammation as the body tries to heal the damage site. Studies have shown that high level of homocysteines is one of the most serious problems for heart disease and increases a person's risk of heart attack by 300 percent. Intake of a little extra B-vitamins, will correct the problem. The discussion in this direction will take us afar.

WARNING

There is another very serious problem for people who are taking statin drugs. According to Dr. David G. Williams, these cholesterol lowering statin drugs are not only ineffective, but potentially deadly. Co-enzyme Q10 (CoQ10) is an extremely important nutrient for maintaining a healthy heart. But what most people don't know is that people taking statin drugs deplete their most essential heart nutrient, CoQ10 that supplies energy for the heart's pumping action, and also help produce ATP to energize the cells.

CoQ10 is Considered as spark plug

Our body have anywhere from 67 to 100 trillion cells depending on
the size of a person.
CoQ10 energizes each cell with the fuel ATP. it produces. Thus, Paucity
or deficiency of coQ10 can lead to serious heart and cell damage, and hence the body.

Next: our heart beats 100,000 times per day. If you make your fist, the size of
your heart is same as that of your fist. People who are obese or overweight,
their hearts suffer a lot, because it has to pump blood to a larger area than it
is designed for.

furthermore, CoQ10 is the most potent heart tonic. Heart needs it to pump blood
properly. It also fuels heart. Without CoQ10 or lack of it, heart will suffer seriously.

We have mentioned above the two most important benefits of CoQ10. But CoQ10 has numerous health benefits like lowers high blood pressure, risk of cancer, diabetes, angina, and heart attacks. Reduces high cholesterol, and improves brain health, and so on.

NOTE: CoQ10 and selenium together improves heart function. These two together reduce mitochondrial (mitochondria are power houses of cells) damage and produce new ones.

For More information on CoQ10 and mitochondria consult the book entitled " **SECRETES REVEALED STAY YOUNG AND HEALTHY WITH LIMITLESS ENERGY"** **By** Dr. Arta Tran Dash, M.Sc., M.S., Ph.D. Published by Kindle Publishing, Amazon.

Studies overwhelmingly have shown that statin drugs produce dangerous CoQ10 paucities that can create heart failure. Ironically, lowering cholesterol through statin drugs is supposed to prevent heart attacks and/or heart failures; instead they produce heart failures and/or heart attacks.

Here is an example: I used to play golf with a doctor friend. In 2017 summer, I did not see him in the club for some time. After a couple of months, I noticed he is hitting balls in the range, but looks pale and rundown. I asked him are you ok? I have not seen you for a while.

He said I had heart attack. The trouble with the doctors, they consider all the natural supplements are placebos, and waste of money. Then I asked him, were you taking by chance taking cholesterol lowering statin drugs? He said yes. I mentioned to him that cholesterol lowering statin drugs deplete the most important heart nutrient CoQ10. The deficiency of this nutrient or lack of it may cause heart attacks.

You see the evidence that scandalous advertisement by greedy drug companies and doctors push statin drugs to patients to prevent heart attacks/strokes is extremely dangerous and ineffective, instead these drugs cause heart attacks and strokes.

If he would have taken CoQ10 300 mg in divided doses. He probably would not have heart attack, if he did, it would be much less severe..

Second Example: President of heart Association had a heart attack diring the conference. I would not be surprised to know that he was taking statin drugs.

Suggestion: If you decide to remain on a statin drug, the only way you can protect yourself is to take CoQ10 supplements along with your statin drugs. See the reference below.

Dose: CoQ10, 100 mg three times daily

Ref: Williams, David, M.D., **Alternatives;** Vol. 31, Spring 2007.

Furthermore, recent studies have shown that cholesterol lowering statin drugs are "making the patients stupid"—literary. After just six months of use the study group showed a marked decline in their mental sharpness as well as their attention span. These facts were reported by various TV channel news.

Ref: CBS Evening News with Kate Courie;

Statins' Mind-Boggling Effects. O'TALLON, III., May 24, 2004.

Statin Dangers: Cholesterol lowering drugs, such as Lipitor, Zicor, induce heart

failure and more. By Sally Fallon and Mary G. Enig, Ph.D.

CHAPTER ELEVEN

However, our approach here is to lower blood cholesterol levels naturally, free of any side effects.

Start with the following

Set more vitamin C. Vitamin C is the main component of collagen. Your blood vessels need to constantly replenish collagen to remain healthy and plaque-free over time. Good food sources include fruits, bell peppers, and broccoli.

For inflammation-fighting you'll have to take additional amounts of vitamin C in supplement form. Recommend dose. 2000 mg twice a day. Take it with food to avoid an upset stomach.

6. Use Supplements to Support Healthy Cholesterol Particle Size. These include:
• A high potency multivitamin with trace minerals, including at least 500 mcg of chromium, 2 mg of biotin and 400 mg of lipoic acid. For most you will take three capsules twice a day.a
• 1000 mg of omega-3 fats (EPA/DHA) twice a day.

* vitamins C (as mentioned avobe), E (you may have in multivitamins), lipoic acid, CoQ10 and PQQ,
• 2000 IU of vitamin D3 twice a day (Some people recommend less -- consult your doctor.)
• 1200 mg of red rice yeast twice a day (careful, this has similar side effects as that of statin drugs).
• 2-4 capsules of glucomannan 15 minutes before meals with a glass of water. Now a days you can find noodles of konjac which helps reduce cholesterol, lose weight, improve blood sugar, etc.
• Broad-range, balanced concentration of plant sterols. You will usually take one capsule with each meal.

Chromium is known to reduce total cholesterol and increase HDL cholesterol levels. Take 200 mcg twice daily. Chromium also regulate blood sugar, and good fo diabetes. Take chromium picolinate.

7. Consider Using High Dose Niacin or Vitamin B3. This can only be done with a doctor's prescription. It is useful to help raise HDL cholesterol, lower LDL cholesterol and triglycerides, and increase particle size.

These therapeutic antioxidant nutrients not only help reduce total cholesterol levels, lower homocysteine and CRP levels, but also help prevent oxidation of cholesterol by eliminating dangerous free radicals.

An Apple a Day Keeps Cholesterol at Bay?

Apples are rich in pectin, a soluble fiber, which blocks cholesterol absorption in the gut and encourages the body to use, rather than store, the waxy stuff. Apple peels are also packed with polyphenols — antioxidants that prevent cellular damage from free radicals.

Regular use of eating apples lower LDL (bad cholesterol) and increase the HDL (good) cholesterol

Oatmeal also helps reduce cholesterol, and lose weight.

Aged Garlic and/or aged Garlic Extract:

It reduces cholesterol levels and raises HDL cholesterol levels. Other benefits are:

A potent antioxidant, antibacterial, antifungal, antiviral, immune booster, liver detoxification, antidepressant, cancer therapeutic, reduce high blood pressure, prevent atherosclerosis, colon cancer, rectal cancer, breast cancer, prostate cancer, lung cancer, used to treat prostate cancer and bladder cancer, also used treat enlarged prostate, cystic fibrosis, diabetes, osteoarthritis, CFS (Chronic Fatigue Syndrome),

In details:

Garlic/garlic extract (allium sativum): Numerous studies have shown that garlic can:

- reduce total serum cholesterol levels and raise HDL levels,
- boost production of "natural killer" cells that combat cancerous tumors;
- boost immune system response, and thus prevent allergies, colds, anemia, and asthma;
- reduce blood pressure, and dangerous blood clots, which cause most heart attacks and strokes;
- improve blood circulation;
- destroy infection causing viruses and bacteria; can kill 60 types of fungi and yeast;
- lower the risk of certain cancers, especially stomach cancer, prevent certain tumors from growing larger and reduce the size of certain tumors;
- reduce atherosclerotic buildups (plaque deposits) within the arterial system;
- help to remove heavy metals such as lead and mercury from the body;
- garlic has anti-fungal and antiviral activities, and it also drastically reduces yeast infection; protect a liver from toxic substances, and rejuvenate/promote a tired liver to normal functioning

Dosage: 300 to 500 mg of aged garlic twice daily.

Primary Natural Therapeutic Remedies

Policosanol:

Numerous research studies have found that policosanol lowers total and LDL cholesterol, Lp(a), and raises the HDL cholesterol level.

Dosage: 10 to 20 mg each evening.

Take policosanol for one to two months. Ask the following questions.

    (a) Have the total blood cholesterol levels dropped at least by 20 percent?
    (b) Is the total blood cholesterol level still above 200?
    (c) Is the ratio of total blood cholesterol to HDL cholesterol greater than 4.5?
    (d) Is the LDL (bad) cholesterol to HDL (good) cholesterol ratio greater than 3?

Note: Use only the policosanol extracted from sugar cane wax. It is more effective than the ones derived from beeswax and yams.

If answer to any one of these questions is yes, add to this program the:

Aged Garlic:

It reduces cholesterol levels and raises HDL cholesterol levels.

Dosage: 300 to 500 mg of aged garlic twice daily.

If after one month conditions improve, continue with the program, otherwise add

Guggulu (*Commiphora mukul)* to the regimen.

Guggulu (also known as **Guggull**) is an ancient Ayurvedic Indian herb which is reputed to be effective in reducing triglyceride and serum cholesterol levels, and raising HDL cholesterol levels.

Dosage: 1,500 mg daily, standardized to 5 % guggulsterone (equivalent to 75 mg of guggulsterones)

It should be taken with warm water or a tea of dry ginger to facilitate its fat scraping action.

Other Health benefits Of Guggulu

- promotes detoxification and rejuvenation
- purifies blood
- helps maintain healthy cholesterol levels already
  within the normal range
- kindles agni (digestive fire)
- promotes weight loss

- relieves arthritic pain
- supports immunesystem
- vibrant healthy skin
- protects from infections
- treata skin problems
- prevents heart diseas
- treats skin problems
- Treats acne vulgaris (dose 500 mg twice daily)

People with liver disease, or diarrhea or inflammatory bowel syndrome should use with caution.

If after another month of use you still have not achieved your desirable goal, then you may add Niacin to the program.

Niacin:

Take Niacin in no flush form (inositol hexaniacinate or IP6) in doses of 500 to 1000 mg three times daily. It reduces serum cholesterol levels and raises HDL cholesterol. Talk to your doctor before taking Niacin.

Another extremely beneficial nutrient is

Essential Fatty Acid (EFA) or **Omega 3-6-9** a perfect blend of flax oil, GLA (gamma linolenic acid) for omega-6, and oleic acid for omega-9: Essential fatty acids or Omega 3-6-9.:improves cardiovascular health by promoting proper triglyceride and cholesterol levels.

Arjuna is an Ayurvedic Indian herb which has been used for cardiovascular health since 2,500 B.C. It can help lower total blood cholesterol level as much as 64 % --After only 30 days of use of Arjuna, people see their LDL (bad) cholesterol levels plummet by an average of 25.6 %, with a corresponding 12.7 percent drop in total cholesterol.

Arjuna has been shown to be highly effective in relieving angina conditions. Although nitroglycerine (a drug) is often used for this condition, its effectiveness is reduced with each use, but Arjuna can continue to relieve angina conditions irrespective of how long it's used. Other benefits:

- improves congestive heart failures
- protects from ischemic heart disease
- keep arteries flowing free and clear
- may fight cancer as readily as bacterial infections
- furthermore it is inexpensive.

.

For more details see "Ayurvedic herb angina fights, heart disease, atherosclerosis and more", later sections, *The Ultimate Cures for Heart Disease. Health Sciences Institute (HSI).*

www.hsibaltimore.com.

www.ayurvediccure.com

Beta Sitosterol

It has been known to reduce cholesterol levels over the last three decades. It effectively blocks the absorption of cholesterol resulting in the reduction of total cholesterol levels. In clinical research, doses of beta-sitosterol between 500 mg to 10 grams per day have been used to reduce elevated serum cholesterol levels.

Again use of beta-sitosterol between 60 (20 mg three times daily) and 130 mg per day have been used in clinical trials resulting in reduction in Prostatic Hyperplasia (BPH) and related symptoms. It also helps improve lipoprotein (HDL , LDL) profiles.

Side Effects: interferes with the absorption of beta-carotene and vitamin E absorption resulting in lower blood levels of these nutrients. In high doses, patients may experience nausea and feeling of uneasiness

Reference

Berges RR, Windeler J, Trampisch HJ, et al. *Randomized, Placebo Controlled, double-blind clinical trial of beta-sitosterol in patients with benign prostate hyperplasis.* **Lancet,** 1995, 345: 1529-32.

Klipple KF, Hiltl DM, Schipp B. *A multicentric, placebo-controlled double-blind clinical trials of beta-sitosterol (phytosterol) for the treatment of Benign prostate hyperplasia.* Br J Urol 1997; 80:427-32.

For detailed description of health benefits of Policosanol, Guggul, Niacin, Arjuna, beta sitosterol, antioxidants and other extremely important healthful nutrients,

Consult the book entitled *"Lowering Cholesterol with Nutrition and Natural Supplements, safely"* By **Dr. Art T Dash, M.Sc., M. S., Ph. D. Retired Professor, Published by AuthorHouse, Call 888-519-5121, also advertised in Amazon**

One Important Note

Remember that the cholesterol-lowering statin drugs don't increase the HDL (good cholesterol) cholesterol levels. Raising HDL (good) cholesterol level is far more important than lowering LDL (bad) cholesterol level.

Reason:

When your arteries get "gunked-up", the HDL (good) cholesterol acting as your mop-up squad sweeps away the bad cholesterol attached to your artery walls.

All the natural remedies we have discussed above not only lower the LDL (bad) cholesterol levels, but also simultaneously raise the HDL (good) cholesterol levels. Unlike drugs, they are adaptogens.

CHAPTER TWELEVE

Some Therapeutic and anti-aging nutrients

Unpasteurized Raw Honey

Raw honey is the concentrated nectar of flowers. It is the only honey that is unheated, pure , unpasteurized, and uprocessed. Raw honey is the most healthiest and has the most beneficial nutrients. It contains an important enzyme, namely amylase, concentrated in flower pollen which helps predigest starchy foods.

Commercially processed honeys that are found in the market are heated and filtered so that they look clear and smoother. When honey is heated, it loses its delicate aroma, yeast, and enzymes which activates vitamins and minerals in the body. Research studies have sown that honey's antioxidant properties are comparable to those of fruits and vegetables.

Because of its numerous health benefits, honey is fondly called the *golden liquid*, and it has a healthier glycemic index (GI). When honey is compared with the same amount of sugar, it gives 40 % less calories to the body and it does not add weight. Honey comprises of sugars like glucose and fructose, and minerals such as calcium, magnesium, potassium, sodium chlorine, sulphur, iron and phosphate, including vitamins C, B1, B2, B3, B6, B5 depending on the qualities of nectar and pollen. Here are some of the medical benefits of honey. Honey

- is nature's energy booster, and a great immunity builder;
- improves allergies, sinus problems, bronchitis and bronchial asthma;
- combats depression, fatigue, insomnia, nervous disorders;
- abates blood pressure, cramps, headaches, and urine retention;
- beautifies and soothes the skin, clears many skin disorders;
- helps digestion and assimilation of foods;
- speeds up wound healing, and is effective in the treatment of ulcers;
- has potent antiseptic and antibiotic, antitoxic, and sedative properties;
- soothes soar throat;
- is effective in countering anemia;

Honey's natural fruit sugars, glucose and fructose play a significant role in preventing fatigue during workouts and are rapidly absorbed into the bloodstream when digested by the body. Moreover, honey is known to keep blood sugar levels fairly constant compared to other kinds of sugars. Try the following:

1. If you are planning to work out, take a spoon of honey that will enable you to go for extra miles.

2. If you are feeling low or lethargic in the morning, take a hot toast with honey spread on it, or use honey in your tea instead of sugar for a refreshing surge of energy.

APPLE CIDER VINEGAR

Diabetes

Daily intake of the ACV tonic delivers dietary fibre and other beneficial nutrients, which are needed for regulating blood sugar levels. Moreover, the acids and enzymes promote better digestion and nutrient absorption, which are generally compromised in many diabetes sufferers.

Professor Carol Johnston, Ph.D. and her associates, Department of Nutrition, Arizona University, have shown that drinking ACV slows the rise of blood sugar after the consumption of a high-carbohydrate meal. Researchers found that ACV powerfully changes the way you digest carbohydrates. As a result, you don't get the blood sugar spikes that trigger diabetes and also your insulin sensitivity greatly improves. The research results were reported in the scientific journal **Diabetes Care** in 2004. More research is warranted. See Johnston, C., Kim, C., Buller; *A. Vinegar improves insulin sensitivity to a high-carbohydrates meal in subjects with insulin resistance or diabetes*. **Diabetes Care,** 2004; 27: 281-282.

Acid reflux (Heartburns)

Acid reflux or heartburn is a condition that is caused when some of the acid content of the stomach periodically backs up into the esophagus. Studies have shown that tonic ACV can abate the condition of heartburn. For further information you are advised to go to Earth Clinic web site. Thus, to relieve acid reflux or heartburn, take the anti-aging elixir or the healing elixir daily.

Hair care

Apply two tablespoons of ACV with a tiny pinch of cayenne powder to bald and thinning areas before rinsing, washing or shampooing the hair.

At bed time, dab a mixture of one tsp of ACV and royal jelly capsule on bald spots and leave it there over night.

Note: frequent use of shampoo may damage your hair. Instead, rinsing with apple cider vinegar will help maintain the pH balance of hair and remove the buildups that may result from the use of shampoos and styling products. It will leave your hair soft, clean, and luxurious.

Make a mixture of 1/3 cup (75ml) of organic raw ACV and a quart (1 liter) of water. Store it in a plastic bottle and keep it in the shower for use. After shampooing your hair, rinse it with the ACV mixture and keep for a few minutes, then wash. This will clean up all the buildups caused by shampooing and styling products, and keep your hair soft, luxurious, manageable.

For More Information On benefits of ACV see.

See:

www.apple-cider-vinegar-benefits.com

Apple Cider Vinegar— Miracle Health System by Patricia Bragg

And my book mentioned above

Rooibos Tea Health benefits

provides a whole lot of health benefits. Most importantly, it:[1,2]

- Protects against cancer
- Reduces heart disease

- Eases inflammation
- It even calms down crying babies!

Most often prepared as a tea, some people like to compare it to green tea. But it's much more powerful.

- Cancer froof your cells, improve heart function, fight deadly inflammation
- Rooibos tea has almost 50 % more polyphenols than green tea
-
- And one of these polyphenols — aspalathin — is *only* found in Rooibos. The Cancer Association of South Africa calls it "a leading source of anti-cancer compounds.
- **Rooibos Reduces Hardening of the Arteries**
- But Rooibos does more than protect against cancer — it's also great for your heart
- . **Ease Inflammation Safely**
- One of the main causes of any disease — from Alzheimer's and arthritis to heart disease and cancer — is inflammation. But thanks to its high levels of antioxidants, Rooibos is a powerful anti-inflammatory nutrient.

The way I make the Rooibus Tea

I cut ginger into small pieces or grate it. Boil it with two cups of water for five minutes, then add rooibus tea bag (you can find in any local health food store) to the boiling ginger water, make sure there is enough water in it. Let it boil for 2 or 3 minutes, then drain it to a cup, sip when it cool down a bit.

Now You have health benefits of both Rooibus tea and ginger tea.

OR YOU can just make Rooibus tea without ginger. Take a cup and half pure water. Put rooibus bag on it and boil. After four or five minutes drain the water to a cup. Wait it cool down a little. Enjoy. It taste pretty good.

Do not add milk or sugar (you may use raw honey). You might destroy it's health benefits. You don't have to use ginger, if you don't want. But ginger has many health benefits.

HEALTH BENEFITS OF GINGER

Note: *Women trying to get pregnant or nursing should not take ginger*

Ginger health benefits are well known:: relieves muscle pain, indigestion, upset stomach, digestive problems, etc.

However, the recent clinical studies have shown that ginger is scientifically shown to help:

* **Dissolve** deadly blood clots
* **Boost Blood Circulation** and cure vericose veins
* **Prevent Painful hemorrhoids,** increase vein health and improves healthy blood flow
* **Improve blood pressure fast** - and keep blood thin and healthy
* **Eliminate joint and muscle aches** - helping you to bend, flex and point
* **Boost energy levels to new heights** and infuse oxygen rich blood to every part of the body
* **Keep you mentally sharp** - putting an end to foggy thinking, memory loss of seniors
* **avoid a heart, brain, or lung disaster...**
* **Significant reduction in cholesterol**
* **increases the strength of heart**
  **A new study has found a combination of two delicious spices ginger and chilli paper
  Cou;d slash your cancer risk**

* **increase energy production in heart-** to enhance pumping within heart cells that is required for optimal cardiac output
and much
Medical report published in *Prostaglandins Medicine* states that ginger significantly reduced cholesterol and thromboxane synthesis (a substance made by platelets that causes blood clot formation and constriction of blood vessels)

It is also reported that **ginger increases heart's strength** . This is is why scientists call ginger a *cardiac tonic agent* because of its ability to increase energy production in heart and to enhance punping within heart cells that is required for optimal cardiac output.

Reports published in *Thrombosis Research* have shown that ginger is an effective anti-coagulant that can literally *melt away* blood clots *which could trigger heart attacks.*

According to the *Prestigious National Institute of Health* ginger administered to coronary heart patients produced a **significant reduction** in blood platelets clumping.
Reference
Health Research Labs

How to Take ginger
there are several ways you can take it
- take skin out and grate it put in curry,
- put it in smoothies
- you can make ginger tea as described above, drain the water to cup, you may also put green tea bag on to the boiling ginger water, you get many benefits of both ginger and green tea.

CHAPTER THIRTEEN

If you practice the following regularly, they will bring you bliss, physical and emotional well being.

MEDITATIONS, LIVE IN PRESEN, CULTIVATE SELFAWARENESS

1. **practice Kriya yoga**, regularly (meditation, pranayama, and Hata yoga). In addition to spiritual upliftment, there are numerous other health benefits of Kriya Yoga. Briefly stated, regular practice of Kriya yoga can help the body (including internal organs) and mind stay young and alert, and bring overall well-being.

2.
   Ref: www.babaji.ca

   www.kriya.org

   www.kriya-yoga.org

   www.kriya-yoga.org/faqs.html

   There are various forms of meditation. Below we describe a few of them. If you practice them regularly, they will bring wholeness to every aspects of your life, such as physical, material, mental, astral, and spiritual.

3. **Live in The Present** (Mindfulness Meditation)**:** What does this mean? We go through three stages of time, past, present, and future. If you try to observe

   yourself at any particular moment, you will observe that you are mostly

   dwelling in the past or being fixated in future, but not in the present. Dwelling

   in the past and being anxious about the future will bring misery, sorrow, anxiety,

   and pain.

   Realize that, past is gone forever, and the future is unknown, but *present is a*

   gift. One does not even know what its next breath is going to be. No body has

   the power to change or reform the past or control the future.

A Sanskrit Proverb: *Yesterday is but a dream, tomorrow is but a vision. But today well-lived makes every yesterday a dream of happiness and every tomorrow a vision of hope. Look well, therefore, to this day."*

Try not to be preoccupied with the future so much so that you forget about the Present. Focus on what you do today and tomorrow will take care of itself. Somehow, it always does.

The present moment is the only moment that one has and one must make persistent effort of living in the **Now. Now** is where we should invest our time in setting goals, making plans to achieve them, dreaming about successes, doing creative visualization, and making head way for achieving material and spiritual success.

There are various ways one can practice how to live in the **Now.**

Describing all of them will take us far afield from the spirit of this book.

However, for the sake of completeness and also to satiate the thirst of the readers for knowledge, we describe a few of them below how to put into practice.

Try to develop **continuous awareness** simply through noticing, observing day-to-day activities, and being aware of thoughts and emotions. Whatever you do, be a witness.

   a. **In everyday life,** practice watching all of your activities during the day as much as you can. For example, every time you walk up or down stairs at home or at work, pay keen attention to every step, every moment, even your breathing. Be totally present into the **Now.**

b. when you are washing your hands or taking showers, pay attention to all the sense perceptions associated with these activities, the sound and feel of water, fragrance of the soap, or shampoo or conditioner, drying your hair and combing, and so on

c. when you are eating, pay attention to all the details, such as movement of fork or spoon carrying food to your mouth, chewing each mouthful, swallowing the food, taste of food, washing dishes, and taking out the garbage, always continue to cultivate this self-awareness.

d. always make a habit of asking yourself; what is going on inside me at this moment? But don't judge or analyze, just watch

e. watch out for any kind of defensiveness; within you. What are you defending? By witnessing it, you disidentify from it.

Understand that problems are illusions of the mind and there is no problem at this moment. When you create a problem---you create pain. Tell yourself no matter what happens, I will create no more pains in myself. Don't you ever think that being in love is painful or problematic. Being in love is wonderful, specially unconditional love, and selflove. Receive in giving. It need not be anything much, but it is important to give it as sincerely as possible, with all your heart. For instance, a simple smile or a simple word is all you need to satisfy the Celestial laws.

Realize intensely that the present moment is all you ever have. Make the **Now** your main focus of your life.

As soon as you honor the present moment, all unhappiness and struggle dissolve, life begins to flow with joy and ease.

Cultivate Self-awareness

That is, play the game of conscious awareness. As you read these lines or are engaged in certain thoughts, allow part of your consciousness to stand back as a witness, watch your mind read these or engaged in thoughts; or you may allow your consciousness to be divided into two parts. One part is absorbed in seeing, hearing, doing, writing, reading, thinking, feeling and another part simply being aware of every thing going on? If you do so, you will experience "bliss" in each moment. The game of "conscious awareness" is the only game worth playing. Every time you remember to play it, you win "bliss," every time you forget to be the witness, you suffer, and lose. Now you know what to do.

Here is another simple meditation

Listen to The Voice in Your Head, as often as you can. Pay particular attention to any repetitive thought patterns, those old audiotapes that have been playing in your head, perhaps for several years. When you listen to that voice, don't analyze, judge, or condemn what you here, otherwise the same voice may come in again through back door.

As You Listen to The Thought, you feel a conscious presence----your deeper self behind the thought. When a thought stops, you experience----a gap of **"no mind"** or a gap between thoughts. In the beginning the gap will be short, a few seconds, but slowly with regular practice the gap will become longer. When these gaps occur, you feel certain calmness and peace inside you.

With practice, the sense of calmness and peace will deepen, you will also feel subtle emergence of joy emanating from deep within. The joy of **Being.**

Note: You can practice these meditations at any time and any where. However, if at any time your are feeling blue and/or depressed try these meditations. They will bring solace to your mind, body and soul.

You could also find a quiet place in your house may be a separate room or a corner of your bedroom and build an altar with photos of people you revered (e.g., father and mother), and/or God and Goddesses you usually worship. Sit on a cushion in lotus or crossed leg position facing East or North, back straight and body and mind relaxed. Take deep breaths seven times. Breathe in the air entering slowly through your nose, then breathe out sharply through your mouth. Each time you breathe in, imagine that you are inhaling calmness, peace, and wellness to your body; and every time you breathe out, think that you are expelling all your problems and worries in your life. Now close your eyes and listen to Your Thoughts, don't judge or analyze. As explained above as a thought stops, you will experience a gap or "no mind" In the beginning, you may try it for ten minutes, then gradually increase it to half an hour or an hour depending on your interest.

Here is another form of meditation that you may try to create a gap (gap between thoughts or no mind). Follow the instructions as given above. Then just watch your breath. You will notice that the breath will gradually slow down and come to a stop; and hence creating a gap. You will also experience bliss or you may create a gap by focusing into the **Now.**

I have given you quite a few different forms of meditation and how to create a gap between thoughts. You may practice one or all of them. If you do them regularly, you will surely experience immense health benefits as regards to your over all wellness, such as body, mind, and soul.

Furthermore, benefits of living in the **Now** are numerous. Beside others, they include prevention of debilitating diseases, makes you look younger, prevents premature aging, extends life-span, improves overall well-being, and spiritual fulfillment, and finally it may lead to **self-realization.**

Babaji's dictum: practice: Love, Truth, and Simplicity (simplicity means living within ones means). Again this does not mean that you will stop working to realize your dreams and desires.

Ref: Marshall Govindan Satchitanad, Babaji Kriya Yoga

www.babaji.ca

Aromatherapy

Certain natural fragrances can stimulate energizing effects in the body. According to Kurt Schnaubelt, Ph.D., founder of the Pacific Institute of Aromatherapy, California, the number one choice to improve alertness is lemon oil. Put a drop on your pillow or use a burner or diffuser. Peppermint and rosemary essential oils are also known to have energizing effects.

According to a report in the British Medical Journal Lancet, when lavender aroma was wafted into the bed rooms of elderly patients at night, they slept "like babies."

Although, some doctors doubt the effectiveness of Aromatherapy, medical researchers scientifically demonstrated that Aromatherapy may produce both psychological and physiological effects. Aromatherapy benefits includes headache and depression relief, stress reduction, sleep improvement, mood upliftment, regulation of hormones, muscle relaxation, immune system's stimulation, stimulation of blood circulation, healing of skin diseases etc.

Ref: www.aromaweb.com/recipes/rafresh.asp

Instead of using chemical Air Fresheners, use essential oils to make Air Fresheners

Air Freshener

Ingredients

- get a 4 oz clean new spray bottle which has not been used previously for any other purposes and set it to a fine mist setting

- **recipe:** blends of essential oils that may be used: **20 drops lime, 14 drops bergamot, 4 drops ylang ylang, 2 drops rose.**

You may tweak this recipe according to your liking

Directions: Fill the spray bottle with 3 oz of distilled water leaving one ounce unfilled so that you can shake the bottle well between uses. Then add the essential oils describe in the recipe above.

Shake well before each use. Mist lightly in the room. Be especially careful not to let the air freshener mist fall into open beverages. If some body is sensitive to strong aromas, reduce the number of drops. For further details see

Ref: www.aromaweb.com/recipes/rafresh.asp

Conclusion: Now you are aware of the both sides of the story. Being empowered with this powerful knowledge will help you decide on a regimen (of course, with the consultation of a healthcare professional) that is beneficial for your health and well being.

Reference

1. Willey JZ, Xu Q, Boden-Albala B, Paik MC, et al. "Lipid Profile Components and Risk of Ischemic Stroke: The Northern Manhattan Study (NOMAS)." *Arch Neurol.* 2009;66:1400-1406.
2.
Ravnskov, U, et al. "Lack of an association or an inverse association between low-density-lipoprotein cholesterol and mortality in the elderly: a systematic review." *BMJ Open.* Revised 21 April 2016.
3.
Undas, A, et al. Treatment of Hyperhomocysteinemia with Folic Acid and Vitamins B12 and B6 Attenuates Thrombin Generation. Thrombosis Research. 1999 Sep 15;95(6):281-288.

4.
Saposnik, G, Ray, JG, Sheridan, P., et al. "Homocysteine-Lowering Therapy and Stroke Risk, Severity, and Disability Additional Findings From the HOPE 2 Trial." *Stroke.* 2009;40:1365-1372.
5.
Lee J, Jacques P, Dougherty L, Selhub J, Giovannucci E, Zeisel S, Cho E. "Are dietary choline and betaine intakes determinants of total homocysteine concentration?" *Am J Clin Nutr.* 2010;91(5):1303-10.
6.
Margreet R. Olthof, Trinette van Vliet, Esther Boelsma, and Petra Verhoef. "Low Dose Betaine Supplementation Leads to Immediate and Long Term Lowering of Plasma Homocysteine in Healthy Men and Women." *J. Nutr.* 2003; vol. 133 no. 12: 4135-413

Bergamot lowers cholesterol

Berberin lowers cholesterol and control blood sugar, but it has some side effect

www.ingramcontent.com/pod-product-compliance
Lightning Source LLC
Chambersburg PA
CBHW081748220526
45468CB00008B/2286